W0227363

CAMBRIDGE LIBRARY COLLECTION

Books of enduring scholarly value

History

The books reissued in this series include accounts of historical events and movements by eye-witnesses and contemporaries, as well as landmark studies that assembled significant source materials or developed new historiographical methods. The series includes work in social, political and military history on a wide range of periods and regions, giving modern scholars ready access to influential publications of the past.

Recollections of Past Life

First published in 1872, this memoir recounts the extraordinary life of Sir Henry Holland (1788–1873), physician, and travel writer. Holland's first voyage abroad was a four-month trip to Iceland in 1810, and he went on to traverse much of the globe by boat, on horseback, and on foot. He journeyed through Europe during the Napoleonic Wars, survived earthquakes and other disasters, and was arrested three times during his travels. Holland was also well known as a society doctor in London, and this work also includes numerous references to the eminent people Holland treated in a medical capacity. He was medical attendant to Queen Caroline, wife of George IV, and was appointed physician-extraordinary to Queen Victoria in 1837. He also treated six British prime ministers. Originally written for his friends and children and printed privately, the book was revised and expanded for publication the year before Holland died.

Cambridge University Press has long been a pioneer in the reissuing of out-of-print titles from its own backlist, producing digital reprints of books that are still sought after by scholars and students but could not be reprinted economically using traditional technology. The Cambridge Library Collection extends this activity to a wider range of books which are still of importance to researchers and professionals, either for the source material they contain, or as landmarks in the history of their academic discipline.

Drawing from the world-renowned collections in the Cambridge University Library, and guided by the advice of experts in each subject area, Cambridge University Press is using state-of-the-art scanning machines in its own Printing House to capture the content of each book selected for inclusion. The files are processed to give a consistently clear, crisp image, and the books finished to the high quality standard for which the Press is recognised around the world. The latest print-on-demand technology ensures that the books will remain available indefinitely, and that orders for single or multiple copies can quickly be supplied.

The Cambridge Library Collection will bring back to life books of enduring scholarly value (including out-of-copyright works originally issued by other publishers) across a wide range of disciplines in the humanities and social sciences and in science and technology.

Recollections
of Past Life

Henry Holland

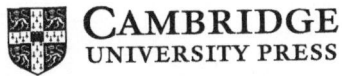

CAMBRIDGE UNIVERSITY PRESS

Cambridge, New York, Melbourne, Madrid, Cape Town,
Singapore, São Paolo, Delhi, Tokyo, Mexico City

Published in the United States of America by Cambridge University Press, New York

www.cambridge.org
Information on this title: www.cambridge.org/9781108038010

© in this compilation Cambridge University Press 2011

This edition first published 1872
This digitally printed version 2011

ISBN 978-1-108-03801-0 Paperback

This book reproduces the text of the original edition. The content and language reflect
the beliefs, practices and terminology of their time, and have not been updated.

Cambridge University Press wishes to make clear that the book, unless originally published
by Cambridge, is not being republished by, in association or collaboration with, or
with the endorsement or approval of, the original publisher or its successors in title.

RECOLLECTIONS

OF

PAST LIFE.

LONDON: PRINTED BY
SPOTTISWOODE AND CO., NEW-STREET SQUARE
AND PARLIAMENT STREET

RECOLLECTIONS

OF

PAST LIFE.

BY

SIR HENRY HOLLAND, Bart. M.D. F.R.S. D.C.L.
&c. &c.

PRESIDENT OF THE ROYAL INSTITUTION OF GREAT BRITAIN:

PHYSICIAN IN ORDINARY TO THE QUEEN.

Hoc est
Vivere bis, vitâ posse priore frui.
MARTIAL.

LONDON:
LONGMANS, GREEN, AND CO.
1872.

PREFACE.

SMALL PREFACE is needed for this little volume, to
explain the origin of the narrative it contains, and
the motives which have led, though not without
some reluctance, to its present publication. Autobiography, where justified at all, may generally
best be left to the discretion of those who come
after the subject of it. The estimate a man
makes of himself, and his concerns in life, is often
a very mistaken one.

The 'Recollections' embodied in this narrative
were first put into writing about four years ago.
This was done at the solicitation of my children,
and several friends, who desired to obtain some
record of a life, already long in its duration, and
possessing a certain interest beyond that personal
to myself, from its relation to many others of
more note in the world. As I saw that a mere
manuscript would not satisfy this desire, I printed
privately a small number of copies, which I was

led subsequently to reprint with considerable additions, finding that many beyond those for whom I originally wrote were interested in the narrative, and seeking to obtain it.

The few copies so printed have long been exhausted; and I have been urged by friends whose judgment I rightly respect, to publish the volume at once, with larger additions than those hitherto made. This, I am aware, is a very old and often abused plea for publication. But in the present instance other motives concurred to justify what indeed may almost be deemed a posthumous act, seeing that I go to the press when already advanced in my eighty-fourth year.

It has been told me—and I welcome the opinion as my best justification—that there is much in this narrative which may be practically useful to those entering upon life, or going through its later stages; and that I should be too nicely scrupulous if halting on a mere question of propriety as to the time of publication. I can only state here, that I shall rejoice if this anticipation be fulfilled.

Another motive influencing me is the knowledge that no one but myself could make the additions that have been suggested, and which from the method of my original narrative require to be interwoven into every part of the volume.

Presuming it likely, from the copies already printed, that the book might be published after my death, I have naturally felt desirous to give it a final form beforehand, and while yet having the faculties needful to do this.

Looking generally at the contents of the sheets as they pass through the press, I cannot but see that there are some things for which explanation is due to those who may be readers of them.

First of these is, the large proportion of the narrative occupied by myself and my personal concerns. This is a rock I saw, and sought to shun; but a general revision of the volume tells me that I have failed in doing so. It was hardly a fault when writing, as I first intended, for my family only; but becomes such when what I then wrote has been thus enlarged and published.

A second matter for which apology may be needful is, the broken and desultory form of my narrative; embarrassing probably to many, distasteful to those who look for a clear and connected story of events. Here, again, I must seek excuse in the limited design with which these 'Recollections' were originally written and privately printed. Were I to compose the whole again, I might be able in some degree to remedy this fault, and at the same time to correct any ana-

chronisms or incongruities arising out of the en-
largement of the volume at successive periods.
But I could not bring myself to undertake the
total remodelling of what was already thus written ;
and I must commit the whole as it now stands to
the good will of the reader.

Some excuse may perhaps be required for the
number of notes appended to the narrative, many
of which, as far as the subjects are concerned,
might have been embodied in it. I was not fully
aware of their amount until the printing of the
volume had already far advanced. But even had
I been so, I should have felt some scruple in
withdrawing them from their present place. The
narrative itself is long enough for its subject ; and
those who are not wearied with it may be led to
cast an eye upon the notes below, as some little
addition to what is related in the pages above.

BROOK STREET :
December 9, 1871.

RECOLLECTIONS OF PAST LIFE.

CHAPTER I.

SOME FORM of embodiment must be given to every narrative of life, however desultory; and though my professional life has been more variously blended with other objects and interests than is usual, I believe I may best make this the foundation of what I am about to write. I have, even from an early age, travelled much and lived much in society; but I have never allowed these collateral interests to interfere with the objects or duties of my profession; and, by what I regard as a singular happiness, I have been enabled so to combine these conditions that nothing has been forfeited by their conjunction.

My narrative then will follow in the track thus indicated, annexing the other incidents of life to those which especially regard my professional course from its beginning to its close. Travel, as I have just stated, holds so large a place among these incidents, that I must necessarily give it some special and commensurate place in what I write of myself. But, nevertheless, here also I

B

shall abstain from any formal narrative. In these days of universal movement over the earth, little that I could say would be new or worthy of relation. I put aside therefore all local description and commonplaces of travelling adventure ; limiting myself mainly to those parts of my various journeys marked by any special incident, or coming into connection with persons or events remarkable in the history of the time.

It is right to say in the outset that this Memoir, as its title implies, is founded almost wholly on recollections. I have never kept a journal of the ordinary events of life, deeming this generally a profitless employment of time, and, in the case of a physician, endangering a breach of professional good faith. Excepting references to my earlier journals of travel for incidents belonging to that time, and other references for dates, all that I relate comes mainly from present memory of the past. From anecdotes pertaining to medical practice I have almost wholly abstained, under the consideration just stated.

This is all I need state in explanation of the matter and method of my narrative. I have sought to define the outline distinctly to myself, deeming this a matter of some moment, where my own personality enters so largely into the subject, and where much caution is needed to prevent its usurping too continually upon what I have to relate. Even under this caution, however, I cannot think it amiss, when writing in my eighty-third year, to preface my narrative by a few words touching the totality of this long life. Such general retrospect every reasonable man must needs make from time to time, even when the remnant has become thus short, and the habits of mind so deeply rooted that little of practical effect can be drawn from the retrospection.

I have much cause to say, on thus looking back upon it, that my life has been a prosperous and happy one. But for the loss—inevitable as time goes on—of many endeared to me by the ties of family and friendship, I might fairly speak of it as untouched up to this moment by any serious misfortune. My health, with rare exceptions, has been singularly good, enabling me to maintain to this advanced age most of the habits and interests of earlier life, even those in which physical activity is chiefly concerned. Except in the single instance of a severe surgical operation, which confined me for some weeks, I have never, in more than fifty years of practice, been prevented from attending to the maladies of others by my own illness. The travels, which taken collectively form so large a portion of my life (a rough calculation would make it more than twelve years) have only once or twice been interrupted by illness; and never marred by any serious accident, though several times menaced by the urgent danger of such.

These travels, repeated every year, while maintaining my health, have had an inexhaustible interest for me. The liberality of an excellent father, and my early professional success, saved me, even from the beginning, from those pecuniary anxieties of early life which so often for a time painfully fret the minds even of those who eventually reach professional fame and fortune. This exemption from pecuniary cares has continued to the end, and enabled me to follow my professional career, and to withdraw from it in the manner most consonant to my wishes. What may well rank higher in the scale of human blessings, my children have never been other than a source of satisfaction and happiness to me.

I may further note it as a fortunate condition in life, that, with one exception hardly worth remembrance, I have been wholly free from any personal controversy or quarrel during this long period of years—a benefit best understood by those who have themselves suffered under such social or professional turmoils. This exemption may have been due to several causes, but chiefly perhaps to those peculiar circumstances in my London practice of which I shall have occasion afterwards to speak.

If I can rightly judge myself, I make this slight retrospect in no ostentatious spirit. Looking around me, and to the various experience my profession has afforded, I have sometimes felt a certain vague alarm in this comparative exemption from the ills commonly besetting life; not due to any deserts of my own, though doubtless peculiarities of personal temperament may have had their share in the result. But on these points, though serving in some sort as preface to my narrative, I have no desire to dwell further.

I was born October 27, 1788, at Knutsford, in Cheshire. If venturing to associate this insignificant fact with the history of the time, I might say that I was born on the very verge of the first French Revolution. Of how many later revolutions of that great country has my long life made me the spectator !—one of them, and perhaps the strangest in all its circumstances, actually in progress while I am penning this paragraph. Concerning the first ten years of my life I can say but little ; nor indeed do I recollect much—perhaps less than is usual in the common memories of childhood. If this be so, it is probably owing to the multiplicity and rapid change of objects which have crowded succeeding years, erasing impressions which a quieter life might have preserved. The field of memory, large though it be in many cases, has yet its limits in all ; and the events of infancy and boyhood come back to myself dimly and without continuity—a straggling one now and then darting through the mist of years, evoked by those strange associations which link together things the most remote in the history of life.

These early years were passed in my native town of Knutsford ; with no other absence than an occasional visit to my maternal grandmother at Newcastle-under-Lyne, and to her brother, Josiah Wedgwood, at Etruria. This admirable man, to whose memory a high public tribute has recently been paid, was endeared to all around him in domestic and social life. Even as a child I received kindnesses from him which I gladly keep in remembrance, and which made my Etruria visits always pleasant to me. Through him I come into family connection with his eminent grandson, Charles Darwin—a long and intimate friendship with whom I have more pleasure in recording than any mere family tie. Whatever be the fate of his doctrines, he has given to the greatest problem of Natural History a new framework and direction of research, which will ever remain a monument of his genius and persevering labours.

A year or two of this first period of life I passed at a private school at Knutsford, learning as much perhaps as such schools generally teach, but this very little. Like most boys of the same age, I had a transient fit of military ardour, fostered by attending the sword exercises of a troop of yeomanry, raised in the town at this time of threatened invasion. I have since seen much of actual military life and battle-fields in various countries, but always looking on them from *without—spectator tantum*—as in these early days of boyhood.

A more tranquil pleasure at this time was that ot frequent visits to my paternal grandfather at the old family house of Sandlebridge, between Knutsford and Alderley. His was an admirable example of old age rendered venerable by all the gentler qualities of human nature. He was the most perfect practical optimist I have ever known. Living on and farming his own land, he put to shame the many sayings, ancient and modern, as to the querulous nature of the agricultural mind. He never could be got to complain of the change or 'distemperature of the seasons.' If a particular season was quoted to him as bad for one crop, he always vindicated it as good for another. I never visit this old and picturesque house of Sandlebridge, now belonging to

me, without some remembrance of him coming to my
mind, either as walking cheerfully over his fields, or
tranquilly smoking his pipe in an arm-chair coeval with
himself. I have added three other farms to this Cheshire property, more than doubling its extent. Though
visiting the place only once a year, it is pleasant to me
to retain the old family farm in my own hands, confess-
ing at the same time that my tastes and habits are
little suited to the condition of a landed proprietor.*

Even in this early boyhood, certain other tastes
showed themselves, which afterwards mingled largely
with the incidents of life. I can recollect the pleasure
I had in exploring the country round Knutsford; visiting the little lakes or meres in this neighbourhood, and
following the windings of the brook which supplies water
to my Sandlebridge mill—the miniature precursor to the
many great rivers whose courses I have since followed.
I made myself also a frequent guide to those who came
to obtain specimens of the Saxifraga Hirculus, growing
on a small detached spot in a marsh close to Knutsford;
—the most southern English locality, as I believe, in
which this plant has been found. Years after, when I
came to look for it on the well-known place, it had wholly
disappeared.

In January 1799, having entered my eleventh year, I
went to Newcastle-on-Tyne, as the pupil of the Rev. W.
Turner; and in the house and under the care of this
excellent man I resided four years. The love of travel,

---

* My cousin, Mrs. Gaskell, who knew Sandlebridge well, has pictured the
place by some short but very descriptive touches in one or two of her novels.

even thus early awakened, has left on my mind several traces of this first journey, made more than seventy years ago. I remember well the interest I felt in crossing for the first time the summit of Blackstone Edge, then a long and hard horse-labour above ground, now accomplished by a few minutes of railroad tunnel underneath. Next came the sight of a tide-river and ships, also new to me; and, a few months later, my first view of the Sea from the edge of the cliff at Tynemouth Castle, to which spot I was led blindfold, to enhance the effect of the sight by its suddenness. I attach a certain sentimental interest to this particular memory, associated as it has become with that of my numerous voyages in after years, and their various incidents of peril or enjoyment. Visiting Tynemouth a little more than a year ago, I stood for a while on the exact spot whence I thus looked on the Sea for the first time precisely seventy years before. A few days afterwards I embarked on a voyage of 5,000 miles to Jamaica. Such relations of time to events are not common in the history of a single life.

I pass rapidly over these four years of boyhood at Newcastle, marked only, as far as I can tell, by a fair amount of bodily and mental activity. There was very little constraint upon me, quiet instruction, and a cheerful home. The knowledge I gained was perhaps somewhat vague and general, but such in kind as to give the appetite for more—an important step in every case in the process of education.

Two short courses on Chemistry and Electricity, by

an itinerant lecturer here, formed my first introduction
to physical science ; a very feeble foreshadowing of what
these two Sciences have now become, but enough to
awaken the interest I have ever since felt in their progress. The nitrous oxide (*laughing gas*) had just been
discovered, and the exhibition of its strange effects, at
which I was often an eager spectator, mixed a little
metaphysical thought, such as might occur to a boy,
with the mere amusement of the spectacle. The wonder
indeed is simply the same as that of common intoxica-
tion, or the innocuous phenomena of dreams ; but the
familiarity of these and other kindred conditions disguises much that bears upon the deepest problems of
mental philosophy.

I may notice here also my many pedestrian excursions
round Newcastle, fostering the tastes which at a later
time I carried with me to the more remote parts of the
world. I have often amused myself by bringing into
comparison events thus widely different in place, time,
and degree, yet all having kindred with the same temperament of mind, passing on from boyhood into adult
age. The neighbourhood of Newcastle was one singularly favourable to these juvenile propensities. The
collieries, with their vast and various machinery—the
Tyne, with its crowded navigation, and its then perilous
opening to the sea—the chemical and other manufactures
(now multiplied fourfold) which already lined its banks ;
—these gave objects to my youthful excursions, the
same in kind as those which still especially interest me.
In visiting the principal coal-mines, I descended and

explored thoroughly one or two of the deepest of them—
those which, under the name of Wallsend, have so long
fed the London fires. My walks, often of great length, led
me also to visit the great iron bridge at Sunderland, and
the more picturesque structure of Tanfield-arch; noted
at that time as the two largest arches in England, now
dwarfed into insignificance by the marvellous works of
modern engineers. The same comparative fate has
attended the old colliery horse-railways of this district,
then regarded with some admiration. Among these
rude wooden railroads, however, was nurtured that
genius of George Stephenson which has since done so
much to change the face of the world. The villages of
Wylam and Newburn, where he passed all the early
parts of his life, were familiar to me in my excursions;
and, comparing dates, I find I must have been often at
Newburn when he was still living there as a common
workman. *Faber ipse fortunæ suæ,* one may well say of
this remarkable man.

One of these excursions comes to my memory as
having been made in the Mayor's barge in the annual
survey of the Tyne by the Mayor and Corporation of
Newcastle. This was followed by a public dinner at the
Mansion House, at which I was a guest—a somewhat
rare festivity for a boy of fourteen. What led to my
being thus honoured I do not remember, but I name it
as the first of a long series of such dinners in after life,
in conformity to a usage which, while fulfilling some
useful purposes, has in its frequency become rather a
heavy tax on English social existence.

Another incident in the early part of my Newcastle life was a visit to Mr. George Taylor at Middleham in Durham. This I note, because here I saw, lying in his cradle, a week only after his birth, Henry Taylor, the author of the finest dramatic poem of our time. More than twenty years elapsed before I saw him again, when I had the satisfaction of aiding him in the first step of his honourable public career. Since that time our friendship has been unbroken.

In 1803, I finally left Newcastle, and went for a year to the school of Dr. Estlin, near Bristol. Here I was placed at once in the position of head-boy; succeeding as such to John Hobhouse, afterwards Lord Broughton, who had just quitted the school. This appointment, coming in exclusion of other boys of elder date there, made me at first some enemies, and led to one or two schoolboy fights; but I kept my ground well in these contests, and the jealousies so created speedily subsided.* My most intimate friend here was Richard Bright, with whom I afterwards travelled in Iceland, and who as Dr. Bright held such high and well-merited place in the medical world. At this school I gained more of classical knowledge than at Newcastle, but still very little of that exact scholarship which is reached (with disputed advantage) at our public schools. What now

---

* The petty incidents of a schoolboy's life are often a whimsical miniature of greater things. In war, the fate of a campaign is sometimes decided by a single bold adventure. At this Bristol school I overcame my first difficulties by challenging two boys to fight at once. The combat, in which I should, doubtless, have been well beaten, was in some way prevented; but such mere act of challenge saved me from all further provocations, and established my position in the school.

renders the reading of the Greek and Latin classics one
of my greatest pleasures was an attainment of later
date, and due mainly to private study. The taste was
fostered by my early travels in Greece, but it has
been ripening ever since ; and I do not mistake my
own mind in saying that I have greater enjoyment
from this source now than at any earlier period of life.
To this subject, however, I shall have occasion to revert
hereafter.

The Christmas vacation of this Bristol school I passed
in London, or rather at Stoke Newington, with Dr.
Aikin, a very old friend of my father. His sister, Mrs.
Barbauld, who lived close to him, and his daughter,
Lucy Aikin, gave a certain literary repute to this then
tranquil village ; since absorbed, like so many others,
into the huge mass of the metropolis. I met in small
parties, at one or other of these houses, several writers
of repute of that day, now almost or wholly forgotten,—
the warm admirers of Mrs. Barbauld's masculine understanding and gentle feminine character. She well
merited this admiration. Of the excellence of her
English prose style it is enough to say that I have heard
it warmly praised both by Mackintosh and Macaulay.
Each specified the 'Essay on the Inconsistency of
Human Expectations' as an example of this excellence.

This was my first visit to London, and sixty-six
years have since elapsed. Having known our great City
through all its intermediate changes, I have some difficulty in recalling its exact picture at that time, and the
impressions made upon me. Madame de Staël's descrip-

tion of it as '*a province of brick*' had not then been
given ; but this was undoubtedly a description well
merited at the period of my first visit to London, and
in truth long afterwards. The newest and best streets
(those north of Oxford Street, then terminating in open
fields) were remarkable only for their unmeaning length
and utter destitution of all architectural character—im-
putations still but partially removed. I went through
most of the *sights* of London as they were then cata-
logued for strangers. It may give some idea of their
comparative paucity and poverty, to say that I was shown
the bald frontage of Connaught Place as one of them.
I have often sought to recall the aspect of Charing
Cross, Pall Mall, Piccadilly, &c., as I first saw these
great thoroughfares ; but the memory of the old has
been gradually obliterated by living for more than half
a century under the growth of the new. I can better
recollect the occasional shooting of the Fall at the old
London Bridge in a Thames wherry,—the little dash of
adventure in this according well with those propensities
of character which showed themselves afterwards in
more distant places and on a larger scale. The picture
too is still before me of the bare and dismal fields lying
outside Tyburn turnpike and Hyde Park Corner—now
covered by two new cities, each rivalling many European capitals in extent and grandeur ; and in the
individuality of the dwelling-houses marking at once the
wealth which created them, and one of the most notable
peculiarities of English domestic life. I have known
foreigners come to London, and quit it without having

even seen these city creations of our own time, still augmenting rapidly under our eyes.

I am not one of those inclined to undervalue the changes which time and the growth of arts and taste have wrought in our great metropolis. I believe these changes, present or in progress, to be greater and more substantial improvements than any other city—Paris excepted — can bring into comparison ; improvement, moreover, only in small part the work of Government, but due infinitely more to the wealthy munificence of corporations, companies, and individuals. The large substitution of stucco for brick, the removal of the taxes on windows and glass, and the increased height and ornamentation of private houses, have made a marvellous change in general aspect; but a change so gradual that it needs a memory of the dreary colouring of the old London streets by day, and of the lurid light of their oil lamps by night, fully to appreciate it.

Much, indeed, still remains to be effected for the well-being of London as a city ; and the faults of ancient construction, as well as of climate and coal fuel, render impossible much that might be desired. But the spirit of the time (greatly embarrassed indeed at all times by the disputes so promptly evoked, on points of taste) is fully awake to the object and its fulfilment. The last ten years especially have been prolific of these improvements. Two hours now passed on the Thames between Lambeth and London Bridge, and in that circle of the City surrounding St. Paul's and the Exchange, will show some of the wonderful changes effected during this period — sights almost unknown indeed to those who crowd the drawing-rooms of the West End, yet better worthy of being studied than many of the objects which our continental tourists rush impetuously, and often ignorantly, to see.

I claim a certain right to this short parenthesis from my long and intimate knowledge of London, and from my having visited at various times every single European capital—many of them so frequently as to be familiar with all that has progressively been done for their embellishment. But I have ever maintained true allegiance to our own great City, and note unwillingly that fashion for depreciating it which has grown up in these days of indiscriminate travel, when hasty impressions, often due to novelty alone, are put down and printed as deliberate judgments. After living in London some sixty years, I would willingly endorse Dr. Johnson's opinion as to this City ; uttered indeed when it numbered scarcely a fourth of its present population, and when individual life was less lost in the crowd of human existence than it now is. Those who depreciate what London has done for its own improvement would do well to read Gay's 'Trivia,' and mark the changes that have occurred since the date of that curious poem —not in size alone, but in all that constitutes the true grandeur of a metropolis.*

---

* I recollect one of Gay's couplets, singularly applicable to the two most recent among London improvements :—

> ' Where common sewers a lulling murmur keep,
> And torrents rush from Holborn's fatal steep.'

I returned to Bristol to complete my allotted year there, and with this my very short school life came to an end. Though I cannot say that I have myself suffered by this curtailment of the common form of English education, and the total omission of a public school afterwards, yet I have thought it well to provide otherwise for my Sons ; and the event has justified me in doing so. It is seldom that an individual case can wisely be confronted with general usage.

When leaving Bristol, I made the journey to Knutsford wholly on foot. Setting out thus with the view of seeing Tintern Abbey only, and the valley of the Wye, the sense of pleasure in bodily prowess urged me onwards to complete the journey as a pedestrian. I refer with some interest to this trifling matter, as the early expression of a particular temperament, which has continued through a long life. Much, indeed, of the philosophy of the human mind, both practical and theoretical, lies in these inborn specialities of character, which time and events may modify, but can never wholly eradicate.

Though not yet sixteen at this time, I was called upon for some decision, conditional at least, as to my future course in life. I can scarcely now say whence the inclination came (possibly from the better promise it gave of voyage or travel at a time when Englishmen were almost wholly excluded from Continental Europe) ; but, whatever the cause, my leaning at this period was to a mercantile life. My father yielded, though somewhat reluctantly, to this wish ; and I became an articled clerk in a great Liverpool house, with the privilege reserved to me, through the friendship of a principal partner, of passing two sessions at the Glasgow University, in furtherance of my general education. These two sessions (1804-5 and 1805–6) virtually decided the course of my future life. I went back indeed to the office in Liverpool in the interval between them; but the suspicion gradually ripened into certainty, that I had greatly erred in this my first independent judgment; and at the close of the second session at Glasgow, I sought and obtained a release from the articles which had bound me to a merchant's desk. It would be well if all mistakes in the great adventure of life could be thus early and easily retrieved.

This decision, which was simultaneous with the choice of medicine as a profession, I have never had a moment's cause to regret. I even look back sometimes, especially during the commercial crises which periodically invade us, with a sort of nervousness at the alternative I so narrowly escaped. This feeling came strongly upon me in 1866 (a year notorious for great commercial disasters), at the time of my penultimate voyage to America; when, passing through Liverpool to the place of embarkation, I found myself accidentally in the street, and on the very spot, where my short mercantile career began and came to its end. It was an emotion almost akin to that created by coming suddenly to a place where at some former time life has been in pressing physical peril. Without predicting what might have happened if I had persevered in this first plan of occupation for life, the contrast must have been a strange one with all that has since actually ensued.

The benefit I derived from these two sessions at Glasgow was not limited to the result just noticed. Though a private student—one of the *non-togati* of the College—I was favourably noticed by several of the Professors (Mylne, Young, Jardine, and Millar), and associated with a class of students for the most part older than myself, some of whom afterwards attained eminence in different positions of life. Within the walls of a College so recently boasting the names of Adam Smith, Hutcheson, and Reid, a body of debating youth was sure to be found ; and the questions of metaphysics and theology, then rife in Scotland, furnished ample aliment for discussion. When Sir Isaac Newton describes philosophy as ' an impertinently litigious lady,' he is giving good reason why she should be eagerly courted by clever youths of eighteen or twenty in a Scotch University, many of them destined to the Ministry of that native Church which was cradled amidst controversies, and has fondled them as a luxury ever since. I recollect well the earnestness and heat of these debates, and the utter unconsciousness that many of the questions discussed had been fully argued by philosophers two thousand years before, and some of them wisely recognised even then as impossible of solution. Voltaire's famous definition of Metaphysics, supposing it had been known to them, would have been speedily put aside by these half-fledged and eager disputants

Among the youths at Glasgow with whom I was thus associated, was one who afterwards attained high and merited reputation as the occupant of Dugald Stewart's Chair, and as the most learned of Scotch metaphysical writers. This was Sir W. Hamilton. Exactly of the same age, we became intimate, and I well recollect our frequent arguments on those subjects which gave occupation and fame to his later life. He died seventeen years ago, after an attack of paralysis. It may be that his life was thus shortened by its devotion to topics requiring intense and concentrated thought. The mind can seldom be turned *inwards* upon its own workings without a sense of confusion speedily coming on, suggesting or compelling a cessation of this effort of reflex consciousness.

I discovered a short time ago, among some old books, two essays which I wrote at Glasgow in connection with these metaphysical controversies—one ' On Liberty and Necessity,' the other ' On the Passions in their Relation to the Intellectual Nature of Man.' It interested me to find in one of these essays the passing discussion of a subject on which I have since much more largely written, viz. ' On Time as an Element in Mental Functions,' showing that this curious topic—too little regarded in its bearing on Mental Philosophy—had even then engaged my mind.* Looking at these papers after the lapse of sixty-five years, I detect in them a certain amount of juvenile pedantry ; yet sufficient thought, it may be, for the age at which they were written. Until now I had almost forgotten their existence.

* *Chapters on Mental Physiology*, ch. iii. and iv.

Another composition during my stay at Glasgow was a translation of the Second Chorus of the ' Œdipus Tyrannus,' in competition for a public University prize. The prize I gained, but not improbably from the scanty amount and quality of the competition. Notwithstanding the eloquent lectures of Professor Young, who had the art of giving a sort of poetical pathos to the niceties of the Greek Grammar, the Glasgow youth generally had slender knowledge of Greek, and little taste for versification.* The commercial genius of the place already lorded it over the academical. My poetical success on this occasion, though pleasant at the time, did not seduce me into the paths of poetry. With one exception, I believe I have never since put two lines of rhyme together; though my travels in Greece brought me, while yet young, under the local seductions of Helicon, Parnassus, and the Castalian Spring, as well as of that fountain of Arethusa, and those fair slopes of Hybla, where Theocritus and Bion poured forth their gentle strains, the Δωρὶς ἀοιδά of Grecian song.

A very different literary occupation, if such it may be called, fell in my way at the moment of quitting Glasgow. Released now from mercantile trammels, six months of interval occurred before beginning my medical studies at Edinburgh. At this time the Board of Agriculture was engaged in completing their valuable

---

* There was one particular lecture in Professor Young's annual course (I think that on the Dual Number) in which he was wont to move himself to tears, by his own eloquence, and the beauty of the passages he cited in illustration. This was irreverently called by the students *the crying* or *greeting lecture.*

series of County Reports; and through the suggestion of my friend Sir John Stanley (afterwards Lord Stanley of Alderley), I was entrusted to draw up that of Cheshire, founded upon a short Report of earlier date. Variously and efficiently aided in this work by those more competent than myself, I completed it within the six months of my vacation. The volume was published in the ensuing year; and I received from the Board 200*l.*, being double the sum proposed—a substantial satisfaction to the pride of authorship at eighteen, even thus prosaically directed.

This, however, was not my earliest adventure in print. Some years before, while yet at the Bristol school, I hazarded a letter to the ' Morning Chronicle ' on some current topic of the day. Though forgetting the subject, I do not forget the surprise and pleasure I felt in seeing it in the newspaper a few days afterwards, nor my satisfaction in making it known in the school. I suppose some such emotion to be usual to all who see themselves for the first time in print, and very frequent therefore in these days of almost universal authorship.*

* It was some surprise to me, at a later time, to see this letter of my boyhood in a Collection of Extracts from the Public Journals published by Cobbett. The name and works of this man are now nearly stranded on the stream of time ; but they long exercised a powerful influence on the public mind in England, due partly to his opinions, but yet more to the hardy simplicity and vigour of the style in which he embodied them. I well recollect the eagerness with which Cobbett's ' Register ' was looked for and read on every day of its publication.

CHAPTER II.

I WENT to Edinburgh, then the medical school in highest repute, in October 1806, when exactly eighteen years of age ; and at this point my medical life may be said to begin. I shall make it, as already proposed, the foundation of my narrative ; but without any close adherence to dates, and blending the incidents of travel, society, and other occupation with those more strictly of professional kind. A large digression indeed I must indulge in even thus early, in reference to one of these objects. Enough of my life has been spent as a traveller by land and sea to warrant some more especial notice of this part of it—of the causes which led me so far to deviate from the ordinary course of a London physician—and of the method and direction of the journeys thus mingling with the other concerns of life. The narrative, if it can be so called, must needs be a very desultory one ; but so, in truth, were the travels themselves. Their chief peculiarity consists in having been thus closely blended with a profession to which, in all other ways, I steadily and successfully adhered.

A fondness for travel, as already mentioned, I can trace back even to the memories of my earliest boyhood. It is more strongly marked in my recollections of the four years I passed at Newcastle-on-Tyne. I have mentioned the excursions on foot or by water, which made me so familiar with the neighbourhood of that town, that I could have mapped it from memory without other aid. Geography, especially in that connection with the physical sciences too little regarded hitherto in our English education, has ever been a favourite study with me.* Even at this early time of life I had a singular pleasure in all that belonged to the Tyne—its tidal changes, floods, and windings—and I was accustomed to pursue even to their sources many of the small streams (the *burns* and *deans* of Northumbrian speech) which run into this river. The phenomena of the tides had a particular interest for me. I well recollect the pleasure I felt in following their flow upwards along these little streams ; marking the points to which they severally reached at spring and neap tides ; and their various conflict with the waters flowing downwards. These juvenile recollections are not effaced even by what I have since seen of the gigantic tides in the Bay of Fundy, at St. Malo, in the Severn, and elsewhere. It is not mere magnitude indeed which gives its interest to these phenomena. The tidal flow, even in its feeblest

---

* A few words more as to the imperfect manner in which Geography is dealt with in English education, both public and private. It cannot be taught, in any proper sense of the word, by mere maps, or a bald and wearisome nomenclature of countries, cities, mountains, and rivers. What is wanted is that these should be intimately blended with the history of the world of nature,' and the history of mankind ; thereby better fixing the whole in the memory, and giving to Geography its true rank among the sciences. The change thus indicated is in progress, but much is still wanted for its full accomplishment.

form, expresses the periodical changes of the great globes of our system, and the action of that mighty Force which pervades all we know of the Universe beyond. Here, as in so many other instances, familiarity disguises the wonder that lies underneath. We look upon the Ocean swell, and the flow of rivers inverted twice a day, without thinking of that mysterious power from which these effects proceed, and are maintained without interruption from age to age. I cannot, however, but anticipate a time when the tides will be regarded not in reference to navigation only, but as a great material Power, unceasingly present, and, through the principle of *Conservation of Forces*, and under the direction of human genius, capable of being variously applied to the mechanical and other uses of man.

This fondness for streams, large or small, has clung to me ever since my youth, and often given express direction to my line of travel. The Danube I have followed, with scarcely an interruption, from its assumed sources at Donau-Eschingen to the Black Sea—the Rhine, now become so familiar to common travel, from its infant stream in the Alps to the ' *bifidos tractus et juncta paludibus ora* ' which Claudian, with singular local accuracy, describes as the end of Stilicho's river-journey. The St. Lawrence I have pursued uninterruptedly for nearly 2,000 miles of its lake and river course. The waters of the Upper Mississippi I have recently navigated for some hundred miles below the Falls of St. Anthony. The Ohio, Susquehanna, Potomac, and Connecticut rivers I have followed far towards their sources ; and the Ottawa, grand in its scenery of water-falls, lakes, forests, and mountain gorges, for 300 miles above Montreal. There has been pleasure to me also in touching upon some single point of a river, and watching the flow of waters which come from unknown springs, or find their issue in some remote ocean or sea. I have felt this on the Nile, at its time of highest inundation—in crossing the Volga, when scarcely wider than the Thames at Oxford—and still more when near the sources of the streams that feed the Euphrates, south of Trebizond.

Of these several rivers the St. Lawrence is that most familiar to me, and that which has left strongest impressions on my memory. If not ministering, like the Nile, to history and imagination by the monuments of past ages, there is a grandeur of nature in its origin and course which comes in compensation for this. The creation, it may be said, of great inland Seas, it passes from one to another under various names ; throws its vast volume over the precipices of Niagara ; pauses awhile in the deep basin of Ontario, and issues thence with that blue transparency of water which gives such marvellous beauty to the Lake of a Thousand Isles. Rapids, magnificent in their impetuosity, again occur at intervals, even to the vicinity of Montreal. No traveller ought to leave America without having descended the St. Lawrence and its rapids from Kingston to Montreal, the latter among the fairest and most prosperous of American cities.* Nor should anyone neglect to see those

* The population of Montreal has more than doubled since I first visited the place. No city has nobler scope for future extension. Whether

grand heights of Quebec, underneath which the river flows in its nearer approach to the sea.

In the confluence of rivers I have always found objects of interest, and even of instruction. Stranded at one time for some hours on a sandbank in the Mississippi, at the very point where it receives the vast and turbid volume of the Missouri, I witnessed such confluence on its largest scale. It might be called a huge struggle for supremacy. But in streams far inferior to these great rivers, the commingling of waters in their various relations of volume, impetus, and angle of direction, presents striking and ever-changing pictures to the eye. Even the diversities of colour give character to these confluences ; showing the various sources whence the waters come, and the strata through which they flow ; and curiously exhibiting the manner in which they commingle, often tardily and as it were reluctantly, into a common stream.

Much more could I say of rivers as giving to travel the greatest charm of landscape, while affording lessons in geology and physical geography invaluable to science. Even the simple brook, followed step by step to its source, illustrates in the windings of its channel, its depths and deposits, and the sections which its banks disclose, many of the grandest phenomena and conclusions of geology. In the poetry of every age the flow of river waters has been a favourite theme—one symbol of the life and destinies of man.

it might not have been better as the capital of the Dominion than Ottawa, is a point still doubtful and debated upon.

Akin to this fondness for river scenery, and not without some similar justification, is the interest I have
always felt in the scenery of Islands, especially when
small, and grouped together by the same natural conditions. Whether of volcanic or other formations, they
often best expound those great physical changes which
have successively altered the relations of land and sea
over the surface of the globe. As the remnants of older
continents, or the projections of new land by forces from
underneath, they form in each case the most impressive
memorials of antecedent convulsion and change. And
naturalists now recognise the value of the information
they afford (the Oceanic Islands more especially), through
their floras and faunas, in aid of those inquiries into
the origin and distribution of species which play so important a part in the science of our day. Mr. Darwin
first taught us to appreciate adequately this method of
research.

The Isles of the Archipelago and Levant, irrespectively even of their names and history, have ministered
often and largely to this fondness of mine for island
scenery. A like interest I have felt in the grand volcanic group of the Canaries, with their monarch mountain of Teneriffe; in the Lipari Isles, with their ever-
living volcano of Stromboli; and in the wonderful
islands, gorgeous with tropical vegetation, which form
the northern boundary of the Caribbean Sea. I have
found pleasure too, though of more sober kind, in frequent
passages among the innumerable pine-covered isles of the
Gulf of Bothnia and the Norway coasts; and pleasure also,

nearer home, in repeated visits to the Channel Islands, to the Hebrides, the Orkney and Shetland Isles, to that whimsical little group of the Scilly Isles, seeming as if torn off from the parent peninsula of Cornwall; and, latest of all, to the Faroe Isles, that wonderful outbreak of volcanic rocks from beneath the ocean bed.

I must quit this topic, however, to return to the incidents of much earlier date. During the four years of interval between Newcastle and the commencement of my medical studies in Edinburgh, my taste for travel testified itself in various excursions, often on foot and alone, in different parts of England, Wales, and Scotland. Among other places, I visited Loch Katrine and Glenfinlas, then solitary spots known only to some stray tourist of the day, who came back enraptured with his discovery. Other places, since made familiar by the genius of Walter Scott, were reached in these pedestrian excursions, for which I had trained myself by early exercise. I have already mentioned one instance of this training; and the habit is one which has served me in good stead in many journeys of later date and in more distant localities.

Strangely have all the fashions and appliances of English travel changed since the time of which I am now speaking. The topic is too familiar to need illustration, else I could bring many curious instances from my own experience. The mail-coach, as devised by Palmer, was brought into use in 1788, the year in which I was born; and forty years sufficed to raise it to perfection in speed and punctuality, though by no means in comfort. Displaced by the gigantic rivalry of the rail and locomotive, all has changed with this change. The average rate of speed on English roads has become four times as great as before. On most parts of the Continent, the alteration effected much exceeds this amount. Those who may have travelled, as I have done in 1814 and 1815, over the sands of Brandenburg and Hanover, at the utmost speed of three or four miles an hour (accidents excluded), or even in the central provinces of France, will well appreciate the difference. These things are an index, among so many others, of the vast changes which half-a-century has produced in all the conditions of human life on the earth—beneficial, I willingly believe, in their totality and ultimate issue, yet involving some present drawbacks, and many mighty and unseen contingencies in the future. The ocean telegraph and the steam-engine by land and sea place Man in a new relation to the globe he inhabits; and connect the different races of mankind under conditions pregnant of change, whatever be its nature or import to human welfare.

My first foreign travel—a voyage to Iceland in 1810, and a residence of four months in that extraordinary island—had at that time much of adventure as well as novelty about it, according well with the temperament of mind I have described. Various difficulties and privations, now partially removed, beset the Icelandic traveller in those days; but the alacrity of youth, and great interest in the objects of pursuit, carried me

through them; without a moment of ill-health to frus-
trate these objects, or mar the pleasure and profit of the
expedition.   Sir G. Mackenzie and Dr. Bright were my
companions in this voyage.   We saw much more of the
island than had been done by any preceding visitors,
and from our protracted stay there, more of its inhabitants, I believe, than most of those who have since
followed us.   This stay indeed had well-nigh been
lengthened from four to fourteen months ; the vessel on
which we calculated for our return having been disabled
at sea, and never reaching the island.   After long and
anxious expectation, with a shipless sea before us, the
days becoming rapidly shorter, and every resource of food
and clothing more scanty, we eventually found means of
escape in a small brig, the only other vessel which visited
Iceland that autumn ; and landed in the Orkneys, after
a fortnight's stormy passage, and a narrow escape of
shipwreck at the entrance of Hoy Sound.   Our arrival
relieved much family anxiety, caused by the return of
the disabled vessel without us.

The method of my narrative, especially as regards the
records of travel, has so little concern with dates that I
may well pass over *per saltum* a period of sixty-one
years, and speak of a second visit to Iceland, but a
few months ago, accompanied by my second Son.   Touching at the Faroe Isles and Berufiord, we reached Reykiavik on August 22—a time too late for much travel,
yet allowing him an expedition to the Geysers, while I
satisfied myself with shorter and less laborious excursions.   Irrespectively of the strange and striking aspects

of nature in Iceland, this singular association of the latest
with the earliest of my many voyages was deeply interesting to me, in its sudden revival of old memories, and
the comparison, as far as such was possible, of juvenile
impressions with those,—matured I would fain say, rather
than enfeebled, by a long intervening life. Of personal
recollections there were none. The generation of those
from whom I had received a kind hospitality on my first
visit to Iceland had passed away, and the yet greater
warmth and kindness of my present reception came from
their children or grandchildren. It was strongly testified
at a public banquet of the Althing or Parliament of
Iceland, then closing its biennial session ; and at other
dinners given me by the Governor and Bishop of the
island. This feeling, evoked by the fact—a strange one
even to myself—of my thus revisiting Iceland after the
lapse of sixty-one years, was pleasantly augmented by
the remembrance of my having brought vaccine virus into
the island at the time of my first visit. In proportion to
its population, no country suffered more severely from
small-pox than Iceland when first invaded by this
pestilence.

The course of this voyage showed me parts of the
island I had not before seen, especially the magnificent
mountains, ice-fields, and glaciers of the eastern and
southern coasts ; some of these Jökulls the scene of
the most recent volcanic eruptions. Various changes,
still progressive, I had to note in the material condition
of the people of Iceland, the result of more frequent
intercourse with the continent of Europe. Some of

these changes, and those especially which concern Reykiavik, I have thought it worth while briefly to mention
in the subjoined note. Iceland, though more frequently
visited than heretofore, is still out of the track of common
travel. Its people is one well worthy of study.*

But to return now to the date from which I have so
widely digressed. In less than two years after my voyage
to Iceland, having recently taken my degree in Edinburgh,
I devoted a year and a half to a larger and more various
scheme of travel, embracing almost all that was then
accessible in Europe—Portugal, Spain, Sicily, the Ionian

---

* The total island, larger in surface than Ireland, had a population somewhat short of 50,000 when I was there in 1810. It has now been augmented to about 70,000. The capital, Reykiavik, has grown in greater
proportion, from less than 1,000 to 2,000 inhabitants—an increase due to
steam communication, a growing trade, the transference hither of the College
of Bessastad, and other minor causes. The new houses, still of timber,
are for the most part better constructed ; and whereas, in 1810, there was
not a single garden, or vegetable of any kind growing in the place, there
are few of the new dwellings which have not a plot of ground before them,
garnished with potato-beds, turnips, or cabbages, and even, in two or three
spots, a currant-bush or strawberry-plant, trying to put forth what may be
called fruit. The nurture of flowers within doors has now become a matter
of familiar interest. These changes, slight though they may seem, are of
no small value to the comfort of the people of this solitary little capital.
The restored Cathedral (in which I witnessed an impressive service of
Ordination by the venerable Bishop Pieterson), the new College, and the
Governor's house, grown out of the old prison, may be called the public
buildings of the place. I recognised and visited several of the houses I had
formerly known ; —among others that of Bishop Vidalin, now inhabited by
my excellent friend Dr. Hyaltalin—a child of three years old when I slept
in his father's church on the shores of the Hual-fiord. The sittings of the
Althing are held in the great room of the College. We were present at the
last of the session, to which the Governor came in form, closing a discussion
of two hours, which, though involving some important points of constitutional reform, was conducted with great decorum throughout.

Isles, Greece, and some other parts of Turkey. In 1814 I published a narrative of the Eastern portion of these travels, relating especially my several journeys in Albania and Thessaly, as the region least familiar to the travellers of that time. Strangely enough, it continues to be so, even to those of our own day, though embracing numerous objects to which the classical traveller, whether poet or historian, might fondly cling.

Again quitting England in 1814, I passed a year in Germany, Switzerland, and Italy, in attendance as physician on the Princess of Wales. This, with the exception of a short tour in France and Holland, a few weeks after the battle of Waterloo, was my last absence from England before settling as a physician in London. These early journeys I shall slightly sketch in the course of my narrative, as belonging to a time when travelling was a very different act from that which it has now become—Nature the same, everything else changed.

But my life as a traveller was far from being closed at the time of my settling in London. During the more than half-century which has since elapsed, only two years occur—(and these devoted to Scotch and Irish excursions)—in which I have not passed two autumnal months in journey or voyage abroad—accomplishing greater distances as nearer objects became exhausted, and finding compensation for growing age in the increased facilities of travel. In the series of these annual journeys, which seldom exceeded the time just mentioned, I have visited (and most of them repeatedly) every single capital of Europe—have made eight voyages to the United States and Canada, travelling over more than 26,000 miles of the American continent—one voyage to Jamaica, and other West Indian Islands—have been four times in the East, visiting Constantinople, various parts of Asia Minor, Damascus, Jerusalem, and Cairo—have made three tours in Algeria, two journeys in Russia, several in Sweden and Norway, repeated visits to Spain, Portugal, and Italy, a second visit to Iceland, voyages to the Canary Isles, Madeira, Dalmatia, &c., and other excursions which it would be tedious to enumerate.

When first settling in London, I was menaced by the opinion, coming to me from friends, and not without justification from prior experience, that this scheme of annual travel would be injurious to me professionally. I have in no way found it so. Had I not been attached to my profession, and had it not happened that my practice lay chiefly among the classes who are absent from London in the autumn, the result might have been different. But my early resolution as to this matter of travel, steadily persevered in, has proved a gain to me through all succeeding life. I have come back each year refreshed in health of body and mind, and ready for the ten months of busy practice which lay before me. On the day, or even hour, of reaching home from long and distant journeys, I have generally resumed my wonted professional work. The new methods of inter-communication since steam and electricity have held empire on the earth, often enabled me to make engagements for the very moment of my return. I recollect having found a patient waiting in my room when I came back from those mountain heights—not more than 200 miles from the frontiers of Persia—where the 10,000 Greeks uttered their joyous cry on the sudden sight of the Euxine.* The same thing once happened to me in returning from Egypt and Syria, when I found a carriage waiting my arrival at London Bridge, to take me to a consultation in Sussex Square; the communication in each case being made from points on my homeward journey. More than once, in returning from America, I have begun a round of visits from the Euston Station.

I mention these trifling incidents chiefly as showing the facility that may be gained of taking up instantly an accustomed occupation, after a total abstraction from it by distance, change of scene, and all that concerns the wonted habits of life. And here I may further notice a certain pleasure I have derived from these sudden and strong contrasts—from including, for instance, St. Petersburg and Algeria in the same autumnal vacation—or a Sunday Lutheran service, with all its picturesque local adjuncts, at Leksand in Dalecarlia (a sight every traveller in Sweden should see), and a high solemnity in St. Peter's at Rome, exactly five weeks afterwards—or in coming to my arm-chair in Brook Street, a few weeks after I had been in the Hudson-

---

* My friend, Mr. Grote, when recording this memorable march of the Ten Thousand, consulted with me as to the probable spot where this cry of Θάλαττα was first uttered, as he did also respecting the topography of Spacteria, when writing the story of the Peloponnesian war. While aiding him with the local knowledge I possessed, I was deeply struck with the minute and exact research he had himself already given to these points; as to every other in his great work.

Bay factories on the Upper Ottawa, visiting beaver-dams, and shooting rapids with Indians in their bark canoes —or, again, in a rapid passage, six years ago, from the pine-forests of the Glommen and Drammen valleys in Norway, to the vine-covered banks of the Douro and Mondego in Portugal. A later and stranger, though not so instant a contrast, was that between the tropical scenery of Jamaica, as I saw it in 1870, and the rude Arctic region of Iceland, where I was travelling but a few months ago.

I might draw upon my memory for others of these sudden changes of scene, which, though attractive to myself, would probably be so to few besides. Nor would many feel the pleasure I have found in the very uncertainty of my manner of travel—in starting frequently without any defined scheme of route, and still more frequently changing in its progress the route I had originally designed. Such changes were made necessary by the state of Europe during my early voyages. Though in some degree modified by increasing age, they have been more or less habitual to me ever since.

One cause of this desultory mode of travelling has been, that until of late years I have generally set out alone, trusting for companionship to the chances my route might afford. Whether wise or not in itself—and I do not seek to vindicate it—this practice has happily had no ill result. Some of these casualties of companionship I count among the more agreeable incidents of life. Often, however, it has happened to me to be alone, in places where solitude was rendered somewhat severe by the hardships or hazards of the road, and by the absence of all aid, were this required. At such times, and even in the more common case of long evenings at European city hotels, I have ever found great advantage in some occupation, embracing subjects and scenes wholly alien to those around me. The articles, chiefly scientific in kind, which during many successive years I contributed to the Edinburgh and Quarterly Reviews—one in the autumn of each year—served me here in admirable stead. I chose my subject before departure (generally one familiar from previous study)— read the work or works to be reviewed—methodised fairly the matter in hand, and wrote the articles at such times and occasions of my journey as accident or mood of mind might suggest; using the sea-voyage, which often came at the end of my yearly travel, to put together the several scraps written on the road, and filling up after my return any gaps left by this desultory method of composition. Such breach of continuity in writing is not without its advantages. Separate parts are often moulded together afterwards better than can be done by continuous composition. And, in revision, the wise maxim of Boileau, 'Ajoutez quelquefois et souvent effacez,' applies to prose as well as to poetry; even in those matters of pure science where human thought and speculation are dealing with the great mysteries of the Universe.

Many whimsical differences of scene and subject arose out of the practice just described. There was some sort of pertinency in writing on the 'Physical History of Man' when within 200 miles of Mount Ararat, and on Humboldt's 'Cosmos' at the foot of the peak of Teneriffe.   But the incongruity became greater in penning part of an article on Modern Chemistry under the shade of fig-trees at the Wells of Moses on the Red Sea —paragraphs of another on Meteors and Aerolites in an Arab hut between Medeah and Boghar in Algeria—and portions of a third on the life and character of Julius Cæsar, when travelling on the Illinois prairies.*   Such contrasts, not unacceptable in themselves, afforded me a substantial benefit, by diverting those moments of weariness, or even sadness, which occasionally occur to every one in remote and solitary travel.   It is a benefit which can only be duly appreciated by those who have tried this method.   Books serve to the sam end ; but, according to my experience, less effectually.   They do not so entirely disengage the mind from objects pressing closely upon the senses from without.   Such separation for a time from the outer world, though little noted from its familiarity, is in itself one of the most interesting facts in mental physiology.

Among the articles thus written, I would single out one as having given me peculiar pleasure in its composition.   This was upon the Mediterranean Sea ; succeeding to another of which the Atlantic had been the subject.   I had ever felt a deep interest in this wonderful inland Sea, as well from its physical features

* To this article, published afterwards in a volume with others, I owe the gift I received from the Emperor Napoleon III. of the magnificent folio print of his *Histoire de Jules César.*

(among which may be counted four active volcanoes), as from the records its shores afford of all the most signal events of ancient and modern empire. My voyages upon it, during a period of sixty years, have been very numerous ; enabling me to say, that there is scarcely a single one among the many islands in this vast sea-basin which I have not either seen or set foot upon. I never visit Gibraltar without fresh admiration of that magnificent strait, which forms the sole ingress from the ocean to these inner seas. The Calpe and Abyla of this passage might well be fabled as the *laborum Herculis metæ.* No traveller ought to enter the Mediterranean without being imbued with the history and poetry of ancient times as well as of those of our own day ; for almost every hour brings him within sight of some scene which have these marks set upon it.

From motives which I do not willingly call selfish, though they had my own comfort in view, I have generally sought, when travelling, to disengage myself as far as possible from the name and character of physician. But this object was not always easily attained ; and I have often been subject to demands which I could not refuse, though sometimes involving personal risk as well as inconvenience. Such was especially the case when visiting and pressed to render medical aid at Samsoon, Trebizond, and other places on the southern coasts of the Black Sea, during the prevalence of a severe malignant fever, which brought much mortality at the time into the houses of European residents as well as those of Asiatics. I could not well refuse this aid, though it involved the sacrifices just stated. At Samsoon indeed it was some compensation, on emerging from these dwellings of sickness, to mount an Arab horse, and gallop over a dozen miles of open country on the road to Amasia, and the rock sepulchres of the old kings of Pontus— this highland air the more delightful from its contrast with the atmosphere I had quitted on the coast.

I shall have occasion afterwards to speak of the professional demands made upon me by Ali Pasha, Veli Pasha, and their Turkish and Albanian subordinates, during my early travels in the East—an absurd mockery of practice, to which the term of ludicrous is the lightest that can be applied. At a much later time, when at Cairo in 1847, I was summoned to a formal consultation with a French physician on the case of Ibrahim Pasha, whom I visited at his palace on the edge of the desert, near the site of the ancient Heliopolis. My observation at this time made it certain to me that his life would not be long continued. He died fourteen months afterwards. This was followed by another consultation in Alexandria, at which I was invited to prescribe for the eldest daughter of Mehemet Ali; without the privilege even of seeing the Egyptian princess whom I was expected to cure, and upon the report of an Italian physician who himself knew little of the case and feared to prescribe for it! My advice (founded on private information of gluttonous eating without exercise) was probably unacceptable, and not likely to be followed.

My several visits to the United States have brought to me patients of very different stamp, to whom it was a pleasant office to render aid, as some partial return for the many and warm kindnesses I have received in that country. Such aid, however, is really little needed, where both the principles and practice of medicine are derived from schools of instruction and a medical literature in no wise inferior to our own.

I have just spoken of excursions on horseback on the coasts of Asia Minor. It has often surprised me to find that I retained the faculty of hard-riding over rude country, even when two or three years had elapsed without my mounting a horse. From the mountain summits not far from the tributaries of the Euphrates to Trebizond—from Damascus to Beyrout—from Jerusalem to Jaffa—pressed in each case by the necessity for speed —I have made journeys on horseback which, sitting in my arm-chair at home a few weeks before, I should have deemed impossible. When visiting the advanced posts of the Federal army in Virginia in 1863, a long and flattering article appeared soon afterwards in a Washington newspaper, describing minutely all the incidents of my brief campaign, and complimenting me especially on my horsemanship—a compliment which I believe to have been due to my horse, a fine charger of General Slocum's, much more than to myself. One of my latest rapid rides was over the country around Tangiers in Morocco, four years ago. But a more curious though less rapid horse exercise was that among the mountains of Jamaica, in the autumn of 1870; where the bridle paths climb or creep through dense thickets of tropical plants, inextricably entangled, and festooned by endless varieties of parasitic vegetation. I have a certain sort of pride in recording among my latest rides one in Iceland of nearly twenty miles, but a few months ago ; impeded not by tropical forests, but by bare and rugged volcanic rocks—the great lava-stream of Havnafiord.

I have never carried many books with me in travelling, trusting to what I found readable in one language or other on the road. Virgil, Horace, Burns, and, since their publication, one or two volumes of Macaulay's 'Essays,' have always, however, been with me—admirable company when alone, and often well substituted for living companions. A little volume of Burns, cherished from long familiarity, was swept overboard by a huge Atlantic wave, during a run from Teneriffe to another of the Canary Isles in a half-decked boat. A good Daughter replaced it by another copy for my next voyage ; but I would rather have lost many things of greater nominal value than this little fellow-traveller of former times.

My ability to undertake these distant journeys has been sustained much beyond my own expectation, or the wonted warranty of life. Eight years ago (in 1861), when wearied by a twenty miles' sultry ride from the Sea of Marmora to Broussa, and obliged from fatigue to relinquish the ascent of the Asiatic Olympus which towers so grandly over that City, making it almost a rival to Damascus, I penned at the moment a note of farewell to these pleasures of distant travel. I called to mind that exactly forty-nine years before, after a day passed in the Vale of Tempe, I had slept at the foot of the

Olympus of Thessaly—a calculation of time gone by, which, coming upon me at a moment of weariness, might well justify doubts as to the future, though I am not by nature prone to such misgivings. These doubts were, in fact, wholly premature in date. They partially disappeared under the charm of a moonlight ride in returning to the Sea of Marmora, and have been more completely annulled by later events. In the years elapsing since this excursion to Broussa, I have travelled through the northern provinces of Spain—visited the head-quarters of the Federal army in Virginia in the heat of the civil war—again visited America in 1866 and 1869—been at Gibraltar and in Morocco, in Norway, Portugal, Madeira, and Dalmatia—accomplished in 1870 a voyage to Jamaica, and some other of the West Indian Islands—and in the present year made that second visit to Iceland which I have already described; still comprising each of these excursions within, or nearly within, the wonted period of two months' vacation.

About my latest voyage to America I may say a few words, more especially because I must needs regard it as the last time of my visiting that Continent. It is in truth matter of surprise to myself, and may well be so, that when on the verge of my eighty-second year, I should have been able, without hindrance or even fatigue, to reach the North-Western States and upper waters of the Mississippi—travelling by land, lake, or river, more than 3,500 miles during the five weeks I passed in the country. Much I must attribute to the fortunate circumstances under which I travelled. The

moment of arrival in America was, indeed, saddened by
a telegram telling us of an afflicting event at home
which deprived me at once of the companionship of
my second Son, who for the first time had crossed the
Atlantic with me. The loss was great in many ways.
But I still had as a fellow-traveller during this long
journey my excellent friend Mr. Evarts, the late
Attorney-General of the United States. He, while re-
lieving me from all that was burdensome in travel,
lightened every part of the road by those intellectual
and other qualities which have already given him high
eminence, and will, I trust, be invoked for still higher
duties to his country. I would willingly also name here
the many other American friends, whose warm hospitalities, now as heretofore, have taken away the toil of
travel, and made America almost a home to me.*

The various travels, thus cursorily denoted, could
hardly have been accomplished had I not been fond of
the Sea, and wholly exempt from all the ills which
belong to it. This has been the case from the earliest
voyages of my youthful days. Whether in calm or
storm (and being often upon the sea about the time of
the autumnal equinox, I have know nmuch of the latter)
I am equally able to carry on all the ordinary habits of
life, and to walk the deck under the heaviest swell of

* During the journey recorded above, we stayed a day at Chicago. It
was my third visit to that wonderful city, the growth. of which I had witnessed from a population of 35,000 to upwards of 300,000 souls. I write
this note just after telegrams have come relating the destruction of half of
this city by fire. Few places could recover from such a stern catastrophe.
Chicago will do so.

the Atlantic, when almost single in the ability to do so
The physical causes of sea-sickness being still in question, I am not bound, nor am I able, to explain this
exemption from it, so valuable to me in every way as a
traveller.* The good gained by temporary removal from
the petty cares or serious anxieties of life is a matter
familiar to many ; but few would be found to quote the
Sea, as I do, as the first pleasant stage of annual relaxa-
tion from labour.

That tedium of long voyages, so often complained of,
I have rarely felt. The large proportion of the time
I pass on deck preserves me from this. It is a life of
open space—without toil or compulsion, pleasantly passed
in walking, reading, gazing on the sea and skies, and
sleeping—which latter word I put into Italics, to empha-
size what I have felt as the most genial of the many
forms of sleep. The faculty of reading and writing in
all weathers has been of singular value to me. When
storms are sweeping the deck of the vessel, I have my
resources below. Of gazing upon the sea I am never
weary. The study of the waves—offering to the mathe-

---

* It has often struck me as curious that so little is said of sea-sickness by
Greek or Roman writers, either in poetry or prose. There are indeed a few
well known allusions to it—ancient medical authors mention the fact, and
the very word *nausea* embodies it. But seeing that the physical suffering
must have been then what it is now, and that their voyages on the Mediterranean unceasingly exposed all conditions of men to this malady, it is
strange there should be so little utterance on a subject naturally provoca-
tive of it. Juvenal recites in his Twelfth Satire the various evils of the
sea, and taunts his friend with the folly of committing life to the winds and
thin pine-planks, but says nothing of this more common suffering. In
another passage, indeed, less fitted for quotation, he explicitly denotes it,
as Horace had done before.

matician, in the theory of undulations, some of his most profound problems—is even to the eye a perpetual source of interest and pleasure ; whether seen under the wildest storms of the Atlantic, or the gentler influence of the trade-winds, or as the κυμάτων ἀνήριθμον γέλασμα of the Mediterranean summer sea. The dark blue glassy surface of the tropical seas, heavily heaving at times from the influence of some remote ocean storm, is another of these spectacles which has singularly impressed me. In American voyages there is a further interest in the displays of the Aurora Borealis, becoming more frequent from nearer approach to the magnetic pole. Night after night I have witnessed this magnificent spectacle ; illustrating to the eye (though still under doubtful theoretical conditions) those great magnetic currents which circulate round the globe, are *simultaneously* disturbed in Canada and Australia, and possibly, or even probably, express phenomena in which other globes than our own have part. Science has much to do in this wide field of cosmical research, and will assuredly do it. The instruments and methods of registration now adopted cannot be barren of result.

The rapid and desultory manner of travelling I have described will show how little of scientific or other research it has been possible to combine with it. In earlier life indeed, when visiting Iceland, Albania, Thessaly, and certain other countries, with more time and definite objects of inquiry, I was able to contribute various materials to their geography, natural history, and literary records. The results thus obtained were published at the time—some of them, indeed, now super-seded by the narratives of later travellers, enjoying facilities which did not exist in the days of my youth. These facilities, as I have noted elsewhere, are not an unmixed good. Things requiring and rewarding research are now often hastily passed by, and length of travel substituted for its better objects and results. If this remark would seem to apply to my own case, I would repeat in self-vindication, that my travels during fifty years have been little other than *excrescences* on a busy professional life.

I have ever felt a singular interest in verifying, through natural features or by other evidences, those unknown or doubtful localities which history has be-queathed to our research. This taste was more espe-cially gratified during my travels in Greece. There was pleasure in dipping my thermometer into the springs which gave name to Thermopylæ, and finding it rise to 104 degrees—and in ascending, directly afterwards, the rugged heights of Mount Œta, by the probable defile which the treachery of Ephialtes disclosed to the Persians. There was pleasure also in seeking to attach their old names to the ruins of the several ancient cities of Epirus and Acarnania, which I visited and examined ; and in defining and following through the profound chasm in which it flows, that dark river of Acheron, to which the Greeks assigned both a real and a mythical existence ;—much pleasure again, though somewhat more vague, in rambling, as I have twice done, over the rocky Isle of Ithaca, seeking to determine or imagine the localities which Homer (I willingly assume his personality for the authorship of the Odyssey), adopted as part of the scenery of this wonderful poem.

I felt the same interest, though it was rewarded by very partial success, in the attempt to discover the exact site of some of the Oracles of Grecian antiquity. The first of these researches was directed to the Pythian Cave at Delphi, which I looked for (as others have done with similar failure), in the lower part of the chasm between the Castalian cliffs. It was not until after my return to England that I found a passage in Justin, minute and seemingly authentic enough in description to suggest another spot for future research. This I have quoted below, for the sake of any of my own family, or others, who may hereafter chance to visit the grand scenery of Parnassus and Delphi.*

My search after the exact locality of Dodona was the most laborious of these undertakings, perplexed by the vagueness of the ancient geography of Epirus, and the want of precise local description. In this case again a closer collation of authorities on my return led me to believe that I had been looking in wrong directions ; and

---

* 'In hoc rupis anfractu, *mediâ ferè montis altitudine*, planities exigua est, atque in eâ profundum terræ foramen, quod in oracula patet, ex quo frigidus spiritus vi quadam, velut vento, in sublime expulsus, mentes vatum in vecordiam vertit.'—Lib. xxiv. c. 6.

What scientific interpretation should be given to the words 'frigidus spiritus' it is not easy to say. If, as may be presumed the 'Οσιοι, or priests, rendered the oracular responses, it is not impossible that carbonic acid gas may have been the agent concerned, notwithstanding the phrases which poetry has applied to the inspirations of the Pythian priestess.

that, if traces are yet remaining of the Temple of Jupiter and the fountain of fire, which, together with its oaks, consecrated the old Dodona, these will be found in some place between the valleys of the Achelous and Aracthus, probably near the great mountain of Tzumerka, one of the Pindus chain. The epithet of δυσχείμερος, which Homer twice applies to it, points obviously to a mountain region. I had been looking for Dodona too far to the west of its probable site.*

The hope of future success here is somewhat encouraged by my having discovered, through similar traces, the site of the ancient oracle of Nymphæum, near Apollonia. This too was described as a *fountain of fire*; and under a general direction to the locality, derived from Strabo and other writers, I was further guided by finding an extensive and thick deposit of asphaltum (mineral pitch) near to the presumed spot, telling me at once the probable origin of the fire of the oracle. This was speedily confirmed by observing in close vicinity numerous fragments of sculptured marbles, lying on the margin of a small circular pool of water, which seemed as if boiling, from the large volumes of gas escaping through it. Knowing well the nature of this gas, I struck a light and applied it to some of the bubbles, kindling a flame which speedily spread itself over the pool, to the great admiration of my Albanian guards;—a flame which disclosed immediately the secret as well as the site of the oracle of Nymphæum.

---

* In the first volume of my 'Travels' (p. 206 et seq.), I have discussed at some length this question as to the site of Dodona.

It is in some sort an offence against classical lore to reduce these mysteries to the vulgar level of coal-gas, even expressed under the learned name of hydro-carbon. But science is harsh in its demands for reality, and ministers very little to the poetry of human life, still less to its superstitions. Julius Cæsar must have passed close to Nymphæum, on his march from Apollonia to the passes of Pindus. But the great Dictator was not a man to halt on his way for the responses of an oracle.

I might give other instances to explain the pleasure and interest of researches of this nature, especially in countries where the localities are thus consecrated by the history or poetry of past ages. Prosecuted in my own case with all the ardour and activity of youth, I might yet have accomplished more, had I been better provided with books of reference on the spot, or with the more various knowledge since acquired. Had Pausanias been in my hands, I might have profited greatly by his guidance in these early Grecian journeys. But during the later and longer period of life, though still gathering up all the information that fell in my way, I have never explicitly pursued other objects in travelling than the maintenance of health, and the pleasures derived from active locomotion, and the novel aspects of nature and of human life. I had already learnt by experience to distrust the hasty and partial conclusions which travellers are apt to form and make public; and this distrust I have strictly applied in my own case, when rapidly running over countries without any plan of serious research. It has, indeed, been forced upon me by the frequent need of retracting or reversing my first impressions, when the same objects at some later time came before me.

While therefore gaining much for myself by these annual *parentheses* in my professional life, I learnt but little that would have been profitable to others. Of my earlier travels in Iceland, Greece, Sicily, and other parts of the Mediterranean, I possess many volumes of copious notes. But during the last forty or fifty years, travelling rapidly, and chiefly over routes becoming familiar to the world, the only records I have kept—and these chiefly for my own future reference to times, places, and persons—have been written after my return from each several journey. By this postponement of the pen my recollections have been pleasantly refreshed, and at the same time *sifted* of those daily trivialities of travel and petty personal incidents which are apt to find place in the daily journal of the most sober traveller. Such manner of record is of course wholly inapplicable to the case of untrodden countries, or where science of any kind is concerned in the result.

In my various travels, and especially those in Europe, I have never admitted to myself the necessity of seeing things because others have seen them. Time and convenience have both been gained by an habitual neglect of the covenanted code laid down for tourists. I found by early experience that a multitude of inferior objects does but embarrass the recollection of those which it behoves the memory to retain. To visit the one or two hundred churches, which are written down for inspection in Italy, is to obliterate or enfeeble the impressions made by those of highest historical or architectural grandeur. Following the tracks laid out for him, the Continental tourist often squanders time in loitering through provincial museums and libraries, gazing vaguely on shelves of books, or cases of ill-preserved birds or beetles ; ignorant, it may be, of that wonderful Museum and Library in the centre of London, which concentrates in one spot the treasures of the globe. On these points, however, I must not speak too exclusively from my own habits and experience. Every man has some method, right or wrong, of his own; and general rules on such matters have little use or pertinency.

During my early days of travel, when less restricted as to time, I made numerous sketches, very inartistic in kind, but which have served as material for a few paintings, and for various prints published in my 'Travels' and elsewhere. Afterwards I dropt the pencil, and have never taken it up again ; a loss of little import, save perhaps in the feebler recollection of places deserving to be remembered. Ordinary sketches, like journals, interest few, and are speedily put aside and forgotten, even by the artist. Photography has now achieved a facile triumph over them.

I have never been a collector even of the ordinary curiosities and mementos of foreign travel. Excepting a collection of minerals, chiefly volcanic, which I made in Iceland (and a few broken remnants of which I at this moment see in my garden), I do not believe I have

brought back twenty articles from my numerous journeys abroad. Half of these, whimsically enough, are
walking-sticks, a thing I have never yet used in my
life*—canes from the Jordan, the Alcazar at Seville, and
Morocco—a stick cut at the tomb of Washington, when
visiting it with the Prince of Wales †—others, half-
fashioned by beavers themselves, from the beaver-dams
on the Upper Ottawa—canes from the Blue Mountains
of Jamaica—and one stick of blackthorn, which I believe
to have belonged to Walter Scott;—these form a sorry
museum, even if adding to them a sabre of refined
workmanship, given me by Ali Pasha, with the recommendation of its having been largely used in taking off
the heads of his enemies. This recommendation, though
lost upon me, had seemingly its weight with others;
since, before leaving Turkey, I was more than once
offered for this sabre a sum much exceeding the value of
its Damascus blade. Though thus poor in mementos
of travel, yet, were I devoid of other pursuits, there are

---

* I might still use the words of Juvenal :

Pedibus me
Porto meis, nullo dextram subeunte bacillo.

† This visit to Mount Vernon here mentioned deserves to be remembered
were it but for the extraordinary group there assembled : the President of
the United States and all the members of his Cabinet; the Prince of
Wales and his Suite ; with numerous other guests, all standing bareheaded
before the tomb of Washington, while a dirge was performed to the
memory of the founder of a commonwealth which at this moment
needs men of equal firmness and virtue to secure its future stability.
Looking to the history of the last hundred years, as regards the relations
of England and the United States, the picture of which I here give the
outline cannot easily be forgotten by those who witnessed it. It happened
to me to be present on two or three other occasions of similar kind, and
scarcely less singular, during H. R. Highness' visit to America.

none I should so much desire to assume as those of a collector, whatever the object of his research. The collector of beetles or moths, of ferns or fungi, is a happier man, *cæteris paribus*, than one who has no such definite object of pursuit. The interest here is one which augments with its gratification, is never exhausted by completion, and often survives when the more tumultuous business or enjoyments of life have passed away.

Besides the more distant journeys which have thus chiefly occupied my autumnal vacations, I have found certain *void spots* in the travelling map of Europe still offering a certain novelty to my shorter excursions. Such are, the magnificent mountain region of the Hautes Cevennes, almost unknown even to Frenchmen at the time I visited it—the extinct volcanic district of the Eyfel—the grand scenery of primitive slate mountains in the interior of Corsica—the northern provinces of Portugal—the southern coasts of the Baltic between Dantzig and Memel, including the *Haffs* with their long sea-banks, the nursery beds, or rather receptacles, of amber through successive ages—and that country of East Friesland, which, without a single charm from natural beauty, retained, when I visited it in 1830, more of curious mediæval age in customs and language than any other region of Europe. But these rare spots of travel are every day becoming more rare; and will eventually be swept away by that flood of change which is fast obliterating all local limits and landmarks, as well as the usages of past times, over the earth.

Though singularly exempt from any actual misfortune

yet has my life of travel involved several incidents of urgent danger. The first was a very narrow escape in the ascent of the great mountain of Snœfell-Jökull in Iceland ; distant little more than a degree from the Polar Circle, and never ascended before. Dr. Bright and two Icelanders were with me in this enterprise. When reaching the height of about 4,000 feet, a profound crevasse arrested our progress, passed only by the discovery in one place of a bridge of congealed snow, lying across it. This was crossed safely in ascending ; but it partially gave way under the greater impetus of descent, and one of my legs went through the slender and fragile snow arch. Utterly unable to move or rescue myself, I was saved by the snow poles of the two Icelanders who had already crossed the crevasse, so used as to drag me out of this perilous position, to which I still look back with a certain nervous feeling ; or, I might rather say, seek to shun the remembrance. The slighter hazards of life may be regarded afterwards with a feeling akin to complacency ; but not those in which the question was a momentary one of life or death.

I have much cause, again, for vivid recollection of the month of December 1812, when I was three times exposed to dangers rapidly succeeding each other. The first was a narrow escape from shipwreck on the rude rocks of the Isle of Sarakino, during a night of winter storm, on my voyage in a wretched Greek brig from Salonica to Zeitoun. A strong gale had carried us out of our course almost to the foot of Mount Athos, the summit of which broke out from amidst masses of stormy and portentous clouds. The short delusive calm of a cyclone ensued ; followed speedily by a tempest of wind from the opposite quarter, driving our miserable vessel upon that group of isles of which Skiathos and Skopelos are accounted the chief. The anchors were un-availing against the hurricane—the captain was kneeling before the picture of his patron saint, and the vessel given up by the crew, who threatened to throw over-board my Turkish courier as the evil omen of the voyage. I prepared as far as I could prepare for the worst. It was the mere accident of drifting closely round a point of rock into a sheltered bay which saved us. The alter-native between destruction and safety was one of a few yards only. This was the Sea so well known to Homer, and from the rocky isles and sudden storms of which he drew some of his finest similes. Even now I never read certain passages in the ' Iliad ' without a flash of memory crossing me of my December voyage in the Archipelago. The storm created by the ἄνεμοι δύο, as described in the 9th Book, and on that same sea, might be taken as a pic-ture of the very cyclone which thus endangered my life.

This peril was followed, two days afterwards, by a very narrow escape from the pursuit of one of the nume-rous pirate vessels, the terror of the Archipelago at this period from their bold atrocities, of which mutilation and murder were common incidents, and a heavy ransom the smallest terror of captivity. Ten minutes of earlier pursuit would have placed me in their hands. Piracy has now been banished from the seas of Greece, but it has transferred itself to the land, with outrages of similar kind, far better organised in their commission than are the means used to repress or punish them. An unhappy event of recent date has rendered this too painfully notorious.

Later in the same month, when travelling on horseback in Thessaly from Larissa to Zeitoun, with no other companions than Turks and Albanians, I was overtaken at night by a violent snowstorm while crossing the chain of Mount Othrys. With the sacrifice of a horse which fell over a precipice, I was saved myself only by the boldness and local knowledge of one of the guides who travelled with me. Even now I hold in vivid remembrance the hours spent on this precipitous mountain ridge under the darkness of a December night, and pressed upon by tempestuous gusts of wind and snow which rendered a frequent halt the sole safety for life.* The tranquil month passed at Athens, in speedy sequel to these various perils, came in very grateful contrast to them. Yet here too our comfort was somewhat impaired by a severity of cold extremely rare in Greece. It was the very winter which destroyed the French army on its retreat from Moscow.

* Connected with this dangerous passage across Mount Othrys, comes the pleasanter memory of my last view of the great Plain of Thessaly, from the Khan of Thomako, on the first ridge in ascending the pass—a magnificent landscape, though seen at this moment under the fitful and gloomy grandeur of the approaching storm. Livy well describes this pass, and the wonderful view from Thaumaci,—so named, he says, *ab eo miraculo.*' The passage is worth notice, as a more *detailed* picture of natural scenery than is common in ancient writers. Neither Greeks nor Romans seem to have studied those combinations of natural features which enter into our conceptions of *landscape*, and are the subject of modern art. Architecture and sculpture gave sufficient glory to the Greeks as a people.

Another though lesser peril of shipwreck occurred to
me on the coast of Finland in 1830, when returning
from St. Petersburg to England; and a similar peril in
1833 near the mouth of the Garonne, in a hurricane
which gained a fatal notoriety from the numerous ship-
wrecks it involved.   Other incidents of danger, more or
less in amount, I might gather from the memory of my
travels ; but I have the same thankful comment to make
on them all, that they passed over without any eventful
misfortune.   One indeed of momentary peril in the
Shetland Isles I will mention in a note below, from its
being whimsically connected with another incident of
very different kind.*   Much as I have travelled by rail-
ways, and especially in the United States, where accidents by rail and river so largely abound, I can remember

---

* Visiting the Shetland Isles in 1840, I heard an admirable sermon in the
church at Lerwick, from the minister, Dr. Barclay.   The following day
this gentleman, with two or three other friends, accompanied me in a boat
excursion to the Isle of Noss, wonderful from the wall-like cliffs with which
it overhangs the sea.   Passing round the rude promontory called the Bard
of Brassa, our boat was caught by one of those gusts of wind which sweep
suddenly and impetuously through these isles, and for some minutes we
were in danger.   All others lost their presence of mind ; but Dr. Barclay,
deemed one of the best boatmen in Shetland, seized the tiller, and, by his
firmness and skill, brought us into safety.   .   .   Fifteen years afterwards,
having been previously translated to a Ministry in the west of Scotland, he
became a candidate for the office of Principal in the Glasgow University,
then vacant.   Lord Murray wrote to me, begging that I would see Sir
George Grey, Secretary of State for the Home Office, with whom the appointment lay.   I did so immediately, and put the matter to him in its
simplest form ; expressing my conviction that a man who could preach
such a sermon on Sunday, and the next day save a boat from being
swamped by his firmness and promptitude, was one eminently fitted for the
government of young men and of a great College.   How far this contributed
to it, I know not ; but Dr. Barclay received the appointment, which he has
ever since held with high honour and usefulness.

none with more serious result than a few hours' stoppage in the midst of a magnificent forest in Kentucky, a spot I could well have chosen for such a detention.

Another American forest incident, which might have been more serious, occurred to me in 1850, during a five days' lake and river voyage from Chicago to Buffalo. While the steamer stopped at one of the Manitou Isles on Lake Michigan for firewood, I wandered alone into the dense forest which covers the Isle; lost my way among the tortuous tracks of the woodcutters; and but for an accidental opening which gave a momentary glimpse of the Sun and thereby directed me to the landing-place, should have been left a prisoner in Manitou till some other vessel touched there. My absence had not been perceived; and the paddles of the departing steamer were already in motion as I rushed down to the beach to save myself from this island prison.

I have several times been among Icebergs in my voyages across the Atlantic, but once only with the slightest cause of apprehension, and generally under circumstances enabling me to survey them with tranquil admiration. Such was especially the case on the coast of Labrador, and in passing through the Strait of Belleisle. The long experience and admirable discipline of the modern Atlantic steamers signally provide against this as against other contingencies of danger, in what may well be called their impetuous passage across this ocean.

Seeing how much and in what various countries I have travelled, I am fortunate in having been three times only the subject of robbery. Two of these instances occurred in Albania, where a portmanteau was stolen from me, containing journals, manuscript maps and plans, sketches, &c. ; and a few weeks afterwards a valuable gold watch and ring entrusted to me by Mr. Foresti, the British Resident at Janina, to convey to his family at Zante. The robber in the first case was the Sovereign of the country, the Vizir Ali Pasha— in the second a Septinsular Greek, who travelled with me as my servant. By a curious coincidence of time, the history of these two thefts was first fully made known to me 48 years afterwards, in one of my autumnal journeys. Descending the Lower Danube towards the Black Sea in 1861, I met in the steamboat an old Zantiote gentleman, a friend of the Foresti family. Wishing to give me proof of this intimacy, he drew from his pocket a gold repeater left him as a legacy by Mr. Foresti, my Janina friend. I surprised him by saying that I well knew the watch, as one that had been stolen from my custody nearly half a century before. This declaration of mine, however startling to him at the moment, was speedily confirmed by his own recollections of the history he had heard of the original theft, and of the recovery of the watch, on the arrest of the culprit for some subsequent offence.

When at Athens, a few weeks later, with my friend the Dean of Westminster, I frequently saw General Church, a name well known in the annals of the Greek revolution. He told me that, travelling in Northern Albania some years before, and crossing the river Viosa (the ancient Aous) at Lundra, one of the Albanians with him denoted this as the spot where a young Englishman had been robbed of his portmanteau many years ago ; admitting further that he himself was concerned in the act, and that it was done by express order of the Pasha. Of the latter fact I had been thoroughly assured even before leaving Albania ; and subsequently through M. Touqueville, the French minister at Janina. The motive I ascertained to have been a belief that I had gained access to hidden treasures, or ancient marbles having their value in money, when examining the ruins of the ancient cities of Epirus ; and that my papers related to these discoveries. The singular circumstance which gave rise to, or augmented, this suspicion I have related in the note below.* The robbery in question, including clothes as well as papers, arrested at once my plans of further travel through some unexplored parts of Northern Albania, the interior of the ancient Illyria. Though still making a short journey northwards to examine the ruins of Apollonia and the mineral pitch mines of this

---

* Happening on one occasion to land at Prevesa from Santa Maura, I found Ali Pasha there, with his Court and a large body of troops. He desired me to accompany him to the ruins of Nicopolis, in this vicinity ; whither we went, attended by some hundreds of his Albanian soldiery. Seating himself on cushions, under an arch amidst the ruins, he asked me to point out some spot where I thought hidden treasure might be found. Almost at random, as I myself told him, and careless as to the result, I suggested a spot close to the remains of the ancient baths of Nicopolis. Excavation was instantly commenced, and produced, a few days afterwards, an earthen jar, containing two or three hundred debased silver coins, chiefly of the Emperor Gordian—utterly valueless in themselves, but interpreted by Ali Pasha as proof that I possessed some clue to similar discoveries elsewhere. A few of these coins which he gave me I still possess.

region, I was obliged to return with all attainable speed to the capital of my nominal protector and actual robber. It was a hard and cheerless journey—three or four Albanian soldiers my sole companions, with scanty change of clothing, and a volume of Goldoni's comedies the only book left to me. Nor was I much cheered on the way by the spectacle in one place of the unburied remains of nearly 700 men, massacred by the Pasha's orders and in his presence a year before. It was by his direction that my Albanian guards brought me to the spot, and on my return to Janina he questioned me with a certain fierce earnestness as to this incident of my journey. Articles from the French journals, expressing horror at the massacre, had been reported to him, and he obviously sought to know the impression it made upon me. He was little satisfied with what I said on the subject, and the interview closed with some abruptness.

At no period have I had any direct connection with the army; and I can even affirm (though far from pretending to boast of it) that I have never fired gun or pistol in my life, either as sportsman or in any other capacity. But it is singular how often my travels have brought me upon scenes of modern as well as ancient warfare. My recollections of the latter embrace, among the battle-fields of Greece only, Marathon, Salamis, Thermopylæ, Platæa, Leuctra, Mantinea, Chæronea, Pharsalia, and Actium; all of which I have visited, and some of them diligently explored.* Sphacteria,

* Travelling almost alone, and in the middle of a severe winter, I could not do more at Chæronea than conjecture from the character of the surface

rendered memorable by the narrative of Thucydides, and the wonderful remains of the ancient Syracuse, each copiously illustrating in their localities the relation of the same great historian, I have also visited with his work before me. No places indeed so thoroughly expound in their present natural features events that happened nearly twenty-three centuries ago. Even the more apocryphal incidents of the Roman siege of Syracuse, with which the name of the greatest experimental philosopher of antiquity is associated, can be brought into curious conformity with the local aspects of the spot.*

But to come from these earlier ages to our own century of war and bloodshed. I twice traversed parts of Portugal and Spain during the great Peninsular War —visited the several military hospitals when crowded with wounded from the storming of Badajoz—heard the bombardment of Cadiz by Soult—witnessed the following year, between Alicante and Valencia, the flight of a Spanish division before the French under General Harispe, and had here a somewhat narrow escape of being taken prisoner myself—rode over the battle-field of Vittoria, while many were still lying

that the famous Theban Lion might hereafter be found there. This conjecture, stated in my 'Travels,' has since been realised.

* When Livy, Polybius, and Plutarch afford no evidence as to the burning of the Roman ships by mirrors, we can scarcely accept this statement on later and inferior authority. But the low wall-like cliff, forming the inside of the entrance to the Lesser Port of Syracuse, suggests at once the position Archimedes might have used for the catapults, balista, &c., with which he destroyed the vessels lying beneath.

The ten extant books of Archimedes, though edited in a Latin translation by Barrow, are too little known even to the scientific men of our day.

unburied there ; and witnessed the arrival in that city
of the thousands of wounded and prisoners from the
three days of desperate battle on the Pyrenees, when
Soult was seeking to relieve Pampeluna.   Some twenty
months afterwards at Naples (many events having
been crowded between) I accompanied King Joachim,
mounted on one of the royal horses, to a review of his
army, when about to depart on his ill-fated march
against the Austrians.   Twice I have been in Algeria
during the French war of conquest there ; on one
occasion joining at Blidah the march of a corps under
Marshal Bugeaud, against certain Arab tribes near
Medeah.   I visited also the French head-quarters at
Constantine in Eastern Algeria—a place wonderful in its
natural features, and, under its old name of Cirta,
bringing back to memory the Massanissa and Jugurtha
so familiar to the reading of our youthful days.*

   In travelling through Holstein and the Danish Isles
in 1848, I saw something of the petty war of Germans
and Danes then going on, since followed on the same
field by events of so much higher import.   At a later
period (in 1863), when 75 years of age, I was an active
spectator—I will not say an actor—in the midst of the
great civil war then raging in America.   At the head-
quarters of the Federal army in Virginia, and with the
advanced division on the Rapidan in front of General

* The valley of Sefsaf on the way to Constantine, still frequented by
Lions, may bring to mind the description of Jugurtha in this noble chase—
' Primus, vel inter primos, ferire leones.'   I visited their accustomed water-
ing-place in this valley, and skirted it again by night, but without any
traces of them.   Two were killed here a few months afterwards.

Lee's army, and still more in the country through which
I passed to reach the army, I saw warfare on its largest
scale of action and devastation. Twice before I had
traversed this part of Virginia, then very different in
aspect—a happy and flourishing country, where the
evils of slavery were mitigated by various social conditions more or less peculiar to this great State. The
contrast of scene, as I saw it in the heat of war, was
saddening to the eye and to the mind. But in a region
so variously favoured by nature, time and tranquillity
will restore what has been lost. The too sudden advance of the Negro to political power may retard this
restoration, but cannot prevent it.

Eight weeks of absence from my own house in
Brook Street comprised this extraordinary spectacle of
American warfare, with much besides of political and
social interest, to which my several preceding visits to
the United States gave me access. Living in the hospitable house of my excellent friend Mr. Seward at
Washington, and seeing much of President Lincoln, I
enjoyed facilities which few travellers can obtain. Mr.
Staunton, then Secretary of War, sent Adjutant-General
Townshend with me to the army of the Potomac; an
accomplished soldier and admirable companion, to whom
the expedition was a luxury, as he had hitherto known
the war only through his heavy official duties at Washington. General Meade, the recent victor at Gettysburg,
was at this time in command of the army. By him, and
the other generals and officers at head-quarters, as well
as those at the advanced posts, I was received with a

F

courtesy which I cannot readily forget. Such interludes
are not common in the life of a London physician. But
I have already confessed to a certain pleasure, whether
rational or not, from these sudden contrasts ; and in the
instance just given, this taste, such as it is, was amply
satisfied.*

I might pen a slight episode to this military part of
my story, by relating an armed repulse in an attempt to
land on the Barbary coast, between Ceuta and Tangiers,
five years ago. I was in company with my two friends,
Dr. Falconer and Mr. Busk, who had it in view to
supplement their observations on the limestone, breccias,
and caves of Gibraltar, by corresponding observation
on the opposite African coast. We were in a Government steamer, and put off in two boats, with others of
the party, to seek a landing-place. When close to the
shore, which rises rapidly by broken acclivities into
mountain heights, we were startled by the sudden ap-
parition from behind rocks and trees of some thirty
Moorish soldiers, half naked as to clothing, but well
armed, and warning us by gestures and vehement
speech to quit the shore. An ineffectual parley ended
in a dozen muskets being pointed at us, and the compulsion of a hasty retreat, consoled only by the strange
picturesqueness of the scene thus ingloriously closed.

* This scene of warfare came into even more immediate contrast with a
tranquil visit, a fortnight before, to my friend W. H. Evarts, at his charming villa at Windsor, in Vermont, on the banks of the Connecticut river.
Three years later this pleasure was repeated, with the addition of an
excursion to the White Mountains in his company ; and again in 1869, on
returning together from our long journey to Minnesota.

The only inconvenience from this frequent proximity to war has been an occasional military arrest, never exceeding, indeed, two or three hours of detention, and in two instances at least yielding more diversion than distress. Sketching in 1812, near Torres Vedras, one of the mountain fortresses of those famous lines which had recently repelled Massena's army, I was very justifiably arrested by a company of Portuguese soldiers, and conducted as a prisoner to the presence of the English commandant of Torres Vedras, at whose house I was actually a visitor at the time, and whose praise I engaged for the poor fellows who had so strictly done their duty. The next year my pencil, despite its very slender pretensions, again brought me into trouble. Travelling through La Mancha, I quitted the high road with one of our party to visit that group of Windmills, famed as the scene of the adventure to which the genius of Cervantes has given a living reality. The French had only just evacuated the country, and suspicion still prevailed of stragglers in the rear of their retreat. While sketching the windmills—a half-finished drawing I still possess—a body of guerilla-horsemen, of the band of Abuelo, rushed upon us, lance in hand, seized my drawing-book, and carried us prisoners to the neighbouring town of La Mota. Here happily we found the rest of the party; and after a short examination before the Corregidor, were set free for our further journey. The scene at the windmills, including the guerilla band, was a picturesque one, and well repaid the detention. It further included the little

town of Toboso, seen three or four miles off across
the plain—a name which the same genius has rendered
almost classical to our ears.

My third arrest, in 1846, was more serious, from
being strangely mixed up with the fate of a poor
Professor of the University of Cracow, whom I accidentally met at Breslau, and with whom I arranged
to travel onwards to Cracow in the same carriage.
Coming from Paris, and, as I discovered, a secret
member of the Polish Committee there, his movements had been well watched; and the nervousness
he showed on approaching Cracow was well justified
by his instant arrest at the outer barrier of the City.
I, as his fellow-traveller, was arrested with him, and
conveyed under strong guard to the Hôtel de Ville.
On the way thither, being alone with him in the
carriage, he implored me to permit the transference
from his pockets into mine of a packet of papers, which
he admitted to be such as might compromise his liberty,
if not, at this time, his life. It was a startling request,
and my first impulse, I confess, was that of refusal.
But the solicitation became more urgent, and time
pressed too closely to allow any nice weighing of points
of casuistry and conscience. I consented to receive the
papers, and, thus dangerously freighted, came before
the Cracow tribunal, which was awaiting our arrival.
Here we were speedily separated. His examination
preceded mine, and I presume there was other proof
against him, as I saw him carried off manacled to
prison—to what further fate I never had the means

of learning. For myself, the explanation I gave, and my passport, examined by the Austrian authorities, soon released me; I was treated with much courtesy, and my brief captivity well repaid by an official as well as private introduction to the Director of the great Salt mine of Viëlitzka, the main object of my Cracow journey. Another point of conscience occurred here, as to the fitness of receiving these kindnesses while treason, as the authorities deemed it, was still lurking in my pockets. But this case merged in the former; and I prevented any other by speedily quitting the City for the salt mines, and tearing and dispersing to the winds the papers which for some hours had been weighing heavily upon me.

A few things I may yet add to this short and scattered outline of my life of travel. One is a notice of the peculiar interest I have always felt in Volcanic countries. Four months in Iceland, an early gratification of this taste, instructed me on a large scale as to the various objects of volcanic research. I have been (and I am probably alone in this) on the several summits of Hecla, Etna, and Vesuvius; and have attempted, but failed by accident, to reach that of the Peak of Teneriffe. I have visited the still active volcanic Isles of the Lipari group and Santorin; and more frequently the extinct volcanic regions of Europe—those of Auvergne, the Vivarais, the Eyfel and Rhine, and of the Roman States. Madeira, Porto Santo, and the Faroe Isles, I may also name among the more wonderful results I

have seen of these volcanic actions, now locally extin-
guished.   With all this it has never been my good
fortune to witness any actual eruption, unless the
chronic action of Stromboli be so called.   Columns of
steam and other vapours, jets of flame and ignited stones,
I have often seen, and lava still heated ; but never *flowing lava*, or other of those more vehement actions by
which old volcanoes are rent asunder, new cones and
craters formed, and islands raised from the depths of the
sea.   There is indeed a certain sublimity belonging to
the unknown time and origin of extinct volcanoes ; but
I would gladly have exchanged this for the single
spectacle of Etna in the plenitude of its eruptive power.
I never read one of the finest passages of Greek lyric
poetry, that in the first Pythian of Pindar, without this
feeling coming strongly upon me.*

The passage is easy from Volcanoes to Earthquakes
—the latter not indeed to be coveted as happy accidents
of travel, yet such as I am glad to have known from personal experience.   The two occasions of this experience

* Taking the largest view of volcanoes (and there are now at least 3co
numbered as existing, in greater or less activity, on the earth), I always
regard them as representing not merely local changes and disturbances, but
as the exponents, in common with earthquakes, of that *molten mass* (so
termed in default of a better name) which astronomical suggestions, geological phenomena, and even surface observations, lead us to believe as
occupying the centre of the globe.   Individual volcanoes may be deemed
the *vents* or *spiracles* for the great furnace underneath us — originally determined as such by some casual reft or opening in the rocky crust above, and
deriving any differences in their volcanic character and products from the
particular rocks through which the explosive gases pass in their exit, and
from the various modes and rates of cooling to which the ejected materials
are exposed.

were somewhat singular. Passing a day at Livadia in Bœotia, at the house of the Archon Logotheti, I had just returned from visiting the Cave of Trophonius, the Hercynian Stream and the Fountains of Lethe and Mercury—spots of classic fame grouped together in this remarkable vicinity. From a mid-day sleep which followed these pleasant toils, I was suddenly aroused by the shaking of the whole house, and by those strange rumbling noises, from without and within, which usually attend an earthquake. The first shock was speedily followed by two others ; suggesting to me, as far as I recollect, rather undulation than vibratory motion, but the whole perplexed by the rattling of furniture, and the strangeness of the sensations experienced for the first time. What is now denoted by an especial name (*Seismology*) had hardly then been accepted as a branch of science ; and the wonderful problems put before us by these wave-like or convulsive motions of the solid crust of the earth, were yet only partially submitted to scientific observation.

My second earthquake was at Medeah, near the upper extremity of the great Chiffa gorge, in Algeria. It was one which shook the whole province, as well as the little mountain town where I was stopping at the time, in a house prone to fall even without this subterranean aid. The earthquake occurred in the middle of the night, and produced a strange scene of confusion and dismay among the inmates of the rude and tottering buildings, the ordinary domiciles of African town life, which surrounded us. For myself it did not better the digestion of a dish of *filet de lion*, on which, in company with two French officers, I had supped the evening before—an experiment in diet not likely to be repeated. The actual mischief done by the earthquake at Medeah was not great, but elsewhere in Algeria the effects were more severely felt.

The most striking picture of devastation I ever witnessed from a recent earthquake was at Rhodes, when landing on that beautiful island in 1857. It concurred with the explosion of a powder magazine in adding a new desolation to the gloomy grandeur of the street of the Knights Hospitallers. The earthquake was that which in the preceding year had spread terror and destruction over every part of the Levant. The eastern half of the great Mediterranean basin has in all ages been singularly the scene of these convulsions, denoting changes still going on within that globe on the crust of which we dwell. Science is now occupied, both on astronomical and mechanical considerations, in defining the thickness of this crust, but hitherto without any assured result.

Seeing how largely the casual incidents of travel, and weather especially, influence the impressions of the traveller, and how different are the personal tastes and temperaments brought to the view of nature, it becomes difficult to find any scale of comparison for the grandeur or beauty of landscape. If called upon at the moment to cite those particular scenes which cling most strongly to my memory, I should perhaps name the view from the ruined theatre of Taormina in Sicily—that of the Peak of Teneriffe in descending upon the valley of

Orotava, vividly delineated by Humboldt—and the first
sight of the city and plain of Damascus, on emerging
suddenly from the rocky region whence the Barada (the
Abana of the Bible) bursts forth to give life and fertility
to this Paradise of the East. Let me add further, also
on the recollection of the moment, the first sight of the
Alps from the crest of the Jura ridge ; and the view
from the summit of Pentelicus, magnificent in natural
beauty, and illustrating on every side the history, the
poetry, and philosophy of ancient Athens. I visited this
spot, for the second time, ten years ago, with my friends,
Dean Stanley and Sir Thomas Wyse—admirable companions in such a locality.

These, however, as I have said, are but the first
momentary suggestions while writing, and I might
easily crowd my pages with endless others, furnished by
the recollections of my travels. The Alps alone would
be prolific of instances. A few only of such scenes I
will notice, as having strongly impressed me at the
time, and still clinging closely to my memory.

Though beauty does not enter into the landscape,
and though the scale of objects can scarcely be called
grand, yet is there an austere and gloomy aspect about
the scenery of the Dead Sea which, irrespectively even
of the Biblical history and physical peculiarities of this
extraordinary lake and its solitary river of Jordan, leaves
deep traces on the memory. The bare and sullen mountains of Moab on the eastern side of the lake contribute
to this character. A certain sombre feeling I had on
the spot still clings to the recollection of it, strangely
associated with another scene very remote in place

and time. When first looking on the Dead Sea, the recollection suddenly came before me of the great volcanic lake of Thingvellir in Iceland, somewhat similar in extent, outline, and the stern aspects of its scenery, though widely different in other features. This association has continued ever since—one of those whimsical instances of mental mechanism which we recognise but cannot explain.

My memory brings before me a very different scenery in the mountain coasts of Asia Minor, which in their total extent, from Trebizond at the head of the Black Sea to the gulf of Alexandretta in the Mediterranean—a sweep of more than 1,600 miles—present a magnificent series of pictures to the eye, associated almost at every point with the histories or myths of remote antiquity, and the literature and arts of Greece. The whole region of Asia Minor indeed, bounded by these noble coasts, offers the fairest field still open to exploration; and I have often wondered that the spirit of adventure and research has not more actively taken this direction. The historian and antiquary, the artist and geologist, will all find here ample material for their study.

I may cite, as another fragment of early travel which deeply impressed me, my visit of two days to the wonderful mountain fortress of Suli, a few years after the bloody subjugation of the Suliotes by Ali Pasha—a war on a small scale as to space, but extraordinary in its scenery of combat, and from the various romantic incidents in its progress, to some of which Lord Byron has given a poetic memory. The cannon with which Mouctar Aga, the Commandant of Suli, saluted my arrival gave echoes back from precipices closely fronting the fortress, but with a chasm between some 1,200 feet deep, through which darkly flows the Acheron of Grecian story. The room in which I slept overlooked, or rather seemed to impend over, this abyss. The present insecurity of travel in these wild mountain defiles of Suli explains their being now so little known or visited. The despotism of Ali Pasha gave a personal security to the traveller which is lost under the feeble frontier rule of Turkey.

Passing *per saltum* to a very distant and different scene, I may mention the waterfalls, rapids, lakes, and forests of the Upper Ottawa in Canada, as among my most picturesque recollections of travel. A twelve hours' voyage in a bark-canoe manned by Indians and Canadian voyageurs, excited by the shooting of rapids, and cheered by the chorus of voices keeping time with the paddles of the canoe ; varied, too, by a dinner dressed in the depths of the forest, with beavers working at their dams hard by ; and ended with a six miles' moonlight drive through the bare trunks of a forest blasted by recent fire—these things all contrasted strongly with the antecedents of a London medical life, quitted but three weeks before.*

Another rapid transition I may make to the scenery

---

* These American forest fires (of which the autumn of 1871 has furnished some fearful records, both from the United States and Canada) are little represented on the European Continent. In this journey up the Ottawa, I passed through ten or twelve miles of forest thus blasted by fire in 1852. The total length of conflagration here was nearly sixty miles, with a breadth varying from local circumstances. Nothing can be conceived more striking than this vast wilderness of gaunt, gigantic trunks, denuded of branches and foliage, and blackly charred by fire.

of the Blue Mountains of Jamaica—one of my latest as well as fairest memories of travel. It was my first view of tropical vegetation in its native clime, under its endless variety of forms, graceful and grotesque—a profuse exuberance, density, and struggle of vegetable life, almost startling to the unaccustomed eye. Such as I saw it in these picturesque mountains and valleys, and under the changing aspects of tropical suns and storms, it is a scenery not easily imagined from mere description, not readily forgotten when once seen.

It would be useless to press the memory further for instances touching objects and impressions far too complex to become matter of fair comparison. Yet I must make a single exception on behalf of the Falls and Rapids of Niagara—a scene rendered familiar to me by five successive visits to the spot. I have seen these wonderful passages in one of the greatest rivers of the world under every aspect save that of their winter scenery; and without adding a word of description, I may bring it in proof of their peculiar grandeur, that they impressed me more strongly on my last visit than on the first—an effect by no means unusual when the objects contemplated are thus vast yet simple in outline and colouring. This last visit was made together with H.R.H. the Prince of Wales. Coming direct from England, and calculating the time of reaching Niagara, I joined the Prince at the very moment when he was crossing the river to the Goat Island, and stepping for the first time on the soil of the United States—an event singular enough in itself, and commemorated by a host of photographers on the spot.

My last journey in America, already mentioned, carried me to the more remote Falls of St. Anthony, on the Upper Mississippi. Swollen as I saw them at the time by autumnal rains, these afforded a spectacle second only to Niagara in grandeur. Much I might say also of the Chaudiere and other great Falls of the Ottawa River were I writing a description of travels instead of a rapid narrative of life.*

This might be the place, if any, in which to speak more in detail of those eight voyages to America, which have enabled me to visit more than twenty of the States, and almost every part of those British provinces in which the name of ' the Dominion' expresses the union now happily attained. But I must refrain from any such stretch of my narrative. The subject is so large in itself, and the American continent now becoming so familiar to travellers, that I could say nothing new regarding the outer aspects and scenery of these great and growing countries. And were I to speak of my personal relations in the United States, it would be merely to crowd a page with the names of the many from whom I have received kindness and hospitalities without

---

* I have not mentioned the Great Geyser of Iceland among these special objects of memory. Though magnificent as a spectacle, and unique among such phenomena from its magnitude and other physical conditions, it is to the eye a *transient object*, and changing in aspect at every moment while the eruption lasts. Perhaps to the imagination, and certainly to the physical student of the phenomenon, its intermittent character gives a deeper interest to the great boiling fountain of Iceland. The sagacity of Professor Bunsen, aided by personal observation, has done much to explain the probable cause of changes thus mysterious in their first aspects, and to indicate other changes in progress, which must eventually bring the phenomena to an end.

measure. Still less should I feel justified in using any
knowledge I may have gained of American political
institutions and public men, to express opinions on this
momentous subject. I have not such entire confidence
in these opinions as to warrant my putting them into
any formal shape. The questions involved are indeed
so vast and various, and so complicated, moreover, with
the changes going on throughout the world at large, that
he must be a bold man who would hazard a prediction
for the next half-century. These several topics, then, I
put aside as beyond the scope of the Memoirs on which
I am now engaged.

One word more, before concluding this Chapter, on my
life as a traveller. In the philosophy of mind few facts
so well deserve notice as those which regard the mental
measurement of time, through the sequence of events.
The month of life often differs greatly from the month
of the almanack; and nothing better illustrates this than
the act of travelling. It expands and multiplies time
by the rapid succession of events crowded into a given
period, and may in this way be fairly said to lengthen
the duration of life. My two months of annual travel
have often given me amusing experience as to this point.
Coming back from long journeys in America or the
Levant, it has required some time in my own arm-chair,
with the accustomed books before me, and listening to
the same histories of symptoms from the same patients,
to bring me to the true measure of the time I had been
absent. But this return of reality could not deprive me
of what had been thus virtually added, and happily
added, to the term of life.

CHAPTER III.

AFTER this long digression upon a part of life distinct from, yet closely commingled with, its more serious objects, I now revert to the latter; repeating what I said in the outset, that I do not seek for any continuity of narrative beyond what may suffice to keep persons and events in some general relation to time. This is needful wheré the active stages of life, both professional and social, have been so far prolonged as to include not fewer than three generations within their scope. The medical practice I have yet retained has sometimes of late years brought under my immediate care the great-grandchildren of those whom I attended in early professional life.*

In the foregoing pages I have been obliged to speak chiefly of myself; and this necessity must still, I fear, give the general colouring to what I write, though somewhat relieved by more frequent references to those with

---

* A memento of this passage from one generation to another occurred to me a few years ago, when Lord Stanley (now Lord Derby, then Secretary of State for Foreign Affairs) happened to be dining alone with me. It astonished him to learn, as in some sort it did myself to relate, that I had frequently attended his great-grandfather (the eleventh Earl of Derby) some forty-five years before. This is one instance, among many others, of a series of family successions with which I have had connection either as physician or friend—often happily as both.

whom I have had intercourse in life. I may preface my further narrative, however, by declining, for reasons already given, all anecdotes purely professional, as well as whatever pertains to my own family affairs; and to this intention, with few exceptions, I shall seek to adhere steadily throughout.

I went to Edinburgh, as already stated, at the close of 1806. I have spoken of my professional life generally as a very prosperous one; and I may carry this comment back even to an early period of my medical education. With the intervention of two winters in the London Hospital Schools, I passed in Edinburgh the three required sessions previously to taking my degree in 1811. My residence there was singularly fortunate in circumstances affording not only present pleasure and profit, but telling in various ways on the prosperity of future life. Edinburgh at this period was justifiably proud of the many eminent persons forming its society. Brougham, Sydney Smith, and Horner had indeed very recently departed; but there remained (taking the names as they occur to me at this moment) Walter Scott, Dugald Stewart, Playfair, Jeffrey, Henry Erskine, Murray, Alison, Dr. Gregory, Henry Mackenzie, Dr. Thomas Brown, Jameson, Leslie, Sir James Hall, Lord Webb Seymour, Brewster, &c.—a society well worthy of being denoted and remembered. It was partially dissevered indeed by the political feelings still strong in Scotland at this time, and now further excited by the sudden advent and singular success of the 'Edinburgh Review' as the organ of one party. Edinburgh had not become large enough to neutralise through other and independent interests the feelings engendered by political rivalry—a rivalry too which involved at that time, much more than it does now, the possession of political power in Scotland.

A minor and more whimsical cause of disruption in the Edinburgh society was the controversy going on between the Huttonians and Wernerians, as they were then called—the respective advocates of fire and water, as agents concerned in moulding the crust of the earth. The basaltic and other rocks clustering round Edinburgh furnished ample local material for discussion. No compromise of combined or successive agency, such as reason might suggest, was admitted into this scientific dispute, which grew angry enough to show itself even within the walls of a theatre. A play written by an ardent Huttonian, though graced with a prologue by Walter Scott and an epilogue by Mackenzie (the author of the ' Man of Feeling'), was condemned the first night—as many persons alleged, by a *packed house* of the Neptunian school. It may be that the play itself was more concerned in the fate that befell it.

Despite these controversies, however, the society of Edinburgh at this time was not surpassed by that of any city of similar rank in Europe. Though merely a student myself in the medical classes of the University, my good fortune made me more or less intimate with all the men whom I have named above, and gave me habitual admission into the several circles of their society. This was especially the case in the third winter

I passed in Edinburgh, succeeding my voyage to Iceland
with Sir George Mackenzie. Foreign travel of any kind
was rare and difficult in those days, when the usurpations
of Napoleon had dissevered England almost wholly
from the rest of Europe. But this Icelandic voyage
gained greater reputation in Edinburgh from the scheme
having originated there, and in a certain connection with
the geological controversies just mentioned. As regards
my own share in this reputation, it was somewhat augmented by a preliminary chapter on the 'History and
Early Literature of Iceland,' which, with two or three other
chapters belonging to more recent time, I contributed to
Sir G. Mackenzie's volume, and which obtained considerable success, due chiefly perhaps to the novelty of the
subject. I may add, however, on my own behalf, that I
bestowed much care on this Introductory Essay, gathering materials for it while in Iceland, and adding to them
from various sources after my return.*

This little inroad into Northern Antiquities brought
me into closer intimacy with Walter Scott ; at that time
known to the world at large only by his poetry, but well
recognised in the society of Edinburgh, even by his
political adversaries, as one of its most agreeable and
accomplished members. I still hold in happy memory
the little suppers (a meal now lost to social life) at his
house in Castle Street, of which he himself was the soul
and spirit ; his countenance, heavy in its ordinary aspect,

---

* The *Historia Ecclesiastica Islandiæ* of Bishop Jonson, the worthy suc-
cessor of Torfæus and Arnas Magnæus, was the work of greatest value to
me in writing this Preliminary Chapter.

kindling suddenly into life and merriment at the racy Scotch stories, which he ever had at hand to point and illustrate the matter of converse, whatever it might be. Many of these, as he told them, might have been transferred almost literally to those wonderful novels which were at this time but in embryo existence. A little political sarcasm now and then stole into his conversation, but rarely if ever showed itself in any harsh or ungenerous personality,—a feeling alien, as I believe, to his nature, though I have heard him accused of it. Frequently too at this period, I saw him when listening with enthusiastic enjoyment to 'Lochinvar' and other of his ballads, set to music and sung to him by Miss Clephane (afterwards Lady Northampton), with the fine accompaniment of her harp. This made a picture in itself. It was the poet revelling in the musical echo of his own poetry.*

These are my early recollections of Walter Scott in Edinburgh. My intimacy with him was renewed at later periods, both in London and at Abbotsford. I passed two days with him at the latter place, at the time when those perplexities of business were just beginning to press upon him, which so deeply affected the later period of his life. His cheerfulness, however, was yet unchanged, and he played pleasantly with the *mask* of the

* Alluding to Walter Scott's poems, I call to mind the delight I felt, on returning from some months of utter seclusion in Iceland, in finding at Inverness a copy of the *Lady of the Lake*, just published—the scenery already known to me from one of my early pedestrian excursions. It was an equal though different form of luxury, after my long and solitary travel in Albania in 1813, to find a copy of the *Rejected Addresses* on the table of an English officer at Zante.

author of 'Waverley,' then pretty nearly cast aside. This was especially the case in my morning walks with him around Abbotsford, succeeding to two hours' writing in his study. My intercourse with him was more distressingly renewed at different times during the long infirmity which ended in his death. I saw him frequently on his way to Italy, at the house of his son-in-law Lockhart—already an altered man in effect of the first slight paralytic seizure, and painfully showing this alteration in the effort to recover the stories and events partially lost to his memory. Such struggle of the mind with its own decay, is a sad spectacle in every case—in Walter Scott it was especially so. It was not possible either to aid him, or to arrest the effort. I saw him again in London on the day of his return from the Continent, and each day of his stay here—in a state of hopeless paralysis and very imperfect consciousness. His wishes, as far as they could be understood, all pointed to Abbotsford. He recovered sufficiently to authorise the removal. He reached Abbotsford, but it was only to die there. His frame was fitted for a longer life than sixty-one, and I cannot doubt that it was shortened by the anxious and compulsory labours of his later years. I possess a beautiful silver vase given to me by his four children soon after his death, their names inscribed upon it. Not one of them now survives. One descendant only is left of the family of Walter Scott.

My intercourse with Dugald Stewart, Playfair, Jeffrey, and Alison was as intimate as the difference of age and position permitted it to be. I have especially the plea-

sant memory of various excursions with Professor Playfair—some geological, to spots marked by the fire and
water controversy among the rocks near Edinburgh—
one, a visit to Dugald Stewart at his country house, near
Linlithgow. Another recollection blends itself with this
visit, of a metaphysical discussion with Mr. Playfair,
carried on beyond midnight in his bedroom—any sense
of presumption on my part lost in the charm of arguing
with one so genial and indulgent, and withal of such
clear and upright thought. The question, if I well
recollect, was that of Cause and Effect—one by which
Edinburgh and the General Assembly of the Scotch
Church had been angrily agitated a short time before,
on the appointment of Leslie to the Chair of Natural
Philosophy. This controversy still dragged on both in
books and debating societies ; embittered and perplexed,
as it has ever been, by its relations to theology and by
the ambiguities of language ; but not on these accounts
the less acceptable to the Scottish philosophical mind.
The volume of Dr. Thomas Brown on this question,
indisputably the best among the many then appearing,
raised him into sudden reputation; and probably led to
his succession to Dugald Stewart in the Chair of Moral
Philosophy. With this excellent and very accomplished
man I lived on terms of intimate friendship. His
virtuous and honourable life was too early ended. His
Lectures survive him, and contain much that has been
appropriated, doubtless unconsciously, by later writers
on Mental Philosophy.

Not only in the Speculative Society, then famed as a

school of oratory for future judges and statesmen, but also in the Medical Society of Edinburgh, of which I was one of the Presidents, these metaphysical debates had become the fashion of the day. Those several old disputed questions, destined to be such to all time, were here, as at Glasgow, handled with all the fervour of youth, not allayed by much knowledge of what had been thought and written upon them ages before. Many must have felt, as I have myself done, a frequent reproof to juvenile conceit in finding all the great mysteries of Man and Nature to have been explicitly handled by the philosophers of Greece and Rome. The definitions and speculations of Aristotle thus directed are often as clear and pertinent as any that have been since propounded.

On the occasion of Mr. Stewart's retirement, a meeting was called of those who had been taught from his Chair, to give expression of their attachment to him. I presided on the occasion. Lord J. Russell, then studying in Edinburgh, spoke with earnestness on the object of the meeting, and moved the address—in what he has recently told me he believes to have been his first public speech. The high eminence of Lord Russell, through a long and active public career, makes it pleasant to me to record this simple circumstance of our connection in youth.

With Lord Jeffrey and Lord Murray the friendships of my early college life continued until the death of these accomplished men—strengthened indeed in the interval by various collateral ties. The former had recently been raised into fame by the success of the Edinburgh

Review. His conversation, always rapid and eloquent, though sometimes too suggestive of effort, gave him a great charm in social intercourse, except to those who feared his quick repartee in argument, or had cause to dread him as a critic. I saw much of .him afterwards in London, and visited him at his pleasant home under the Costorphine Hills, a place he made most agreeable to his guests.

Of Lockhart, then a youth like myself, I saw little at this time. I lived with him afterwards in London on terms of intimate friendship ; and painfully witnessed in later years the premature decay incident to a disappointed and often harassed life. He was too sensitive to be the editor of a great Review, dealing with the equally sensitive elements of the political and literary world. He felt the slavery more than the power of this position.

The female side of the society of Edinburgh at this time deserves also some mention. In two or three houses of note, as that of Mrs. Fletcher, it took an exclusively political aspect ; but in others, as those of Mrs. Elizabeth Hamilton, Mrs. Apreece (afterwards Lady Davy), Mrs. Grant of Laggan, &c., the literary and scientific celebrities of the place were well blended with those of other kind. I had the advantage, especially during my last year in Edinburgh, of intimate admission to these several parties. Those of Mrs. Apreece gained for a time a mastery over all others. Coming suddenly to the Scotch capital as a young and wealthy widow—with the reputation and fashions of a Conti-

nental traveller, at a time when few had travelled at all
—acquainted with Madame de Staël, and vaguely reported to be the original of Corinne, then fresh in fame
—this lady made herself immediately a circle of her
own, and vivified it with certain usages new to the habits
of Edinburgh life. A stranger to local politics, her
parties were largely frequented by the fashion as well
as learning of the city, and admission to them eagerly
coveted even by the graver departments of science.
The story was current of a venerable Professor seen
stooping down in the street to adjust the lacing of her
boot. My relations of intimacy with her, begun here,
were continued after her marriage with Sir H. Davy—
a union productive of little happiness—and ended only
with her death.

These fortunate conditions of my Edinburgh college
life occurred chiefly, as I have said, during the later
periods of my residence there. Two years of interval
after my first session were passed partly in the London
Hospitals (Guy's and St. Thomas's), partly in private
professional study. I refrain from any details as to
these several places and courses of medical education.
I went through the accustomed routine of lectures, de-
monstrations, clinical practice, and the less profitable
teaching of books—learning at a later period, for it requires time for the lesson, that actual experience, with a
sense of responsibility attached to it, is the sole school
in which to make a good physician. One of the most
learned men I ever knew in the literature of medicine,
as well as in physical science, was one of the worst prac-

titioners ; borrowing his diagnosis from books, and not from that happier faculty, almost an instinct, which enables some men to interpret and act upon signs which no book can describe. Various improvements may doubtless be made in the methods of medical education : but the subjects in themselves are so subtle and complex, and so blended with the diversities of human character, that no teaching can be really effectual which does not include a certain amount of personal experience and responsibility, conjoined with the talent for comprehending and applying its results.

During this interval, before returning to Edinburgh, I made two excursions to Ireland ; the first of which—a pedestrian tour in the Wicklow mountains—I described in a paper or papers in some periodical of that time, the name of which I now forget. The second (in 1809) was made interesting to me by a visit to Edgeworthtown, then the residence of a large and happy family, of whom few now survive. Mrs. Edgeworth, the mother of many children, and the admirable stepmother of many more, died but four years ago, in her ninety-third year. The friendship I formed with Maria Edgeworth in this my early youth, was continued by frequent meetings in London, and once again at Edgeworthtown, whither I took my two Sons with me. It was still further maintained by an unbroken and affectionate correspondence for more than forty years. Her letters to me would in themselves have formed a volume. One of the last she ever wrote was after reading the first volumes of Macaulay's 'History.' I showed it to Lord Macaulay, who was so much struck with its discrimination and ability that he begged me to let him keep it. A few days afterwards a letter came from her family to tell me of her death !

The house at Edgeworthtown, on my first visit there, curiously betokened the mechanical genius of its master. It was full of contrivances for making the ordinary acts of household life serve to other and unforeseen uses. The mere opening and shutting of certain doors set into motion machinery for winding up clocks, or raising weights in other parts of the house. Mr. Edgeworth showed me another practical faculty he had of adapting his functions as a Magistrate to the genius of the Irish peasantry. Sitting with him in some of his examinations, he elicited on my behalf various stories and bulls which might have found place in some of his daughter's best Irish tales. He had himself certain strong peculiarities of character, and was not popular out of his own family, but loved and respected within it. The history of his four marriages, of which he once himself gave me a summary, forms a curious piece of family biography.

These early excursions to Ireland have been followed by many succeeding visits (I believe not fewer than ten or twelve) to that country, of which I know intimately every part. I have, therefore, some personal justification in expressing my earnest wish that the *impetus* of travel, ever dominant in Englishmen, were more largely directed towards Ireland. An integral and important part of the Empire—its Capital now only twelve hours' journey from London — its fine mountain and lake scenery easily reached in two days—it is a country in a state of comparative isolation. A few hasty summer tours to Killarney cannot be admitted in contradiction of this statement. I have often been amazed by the acknowledgment of able and intelligent men, even members of Cabinets or of the Imperial Legislature, that they had never set foot on Irish soil—an admission made needless, indeed, by their ignorance of the most common aspects and localities of the country. France, Germany, and Italy are annually traversed in all directions; Switzerland is known to its innermost mountain recesses and mountain summits ; even Spain is opening its gates to English tourists — while Ireland continues in some sort a *terra incognita* in the map of travel.

I have no concern here with matters of general policy, with those questions of Church and Land which still agitate and afflict that country, and render Irish legislation as difficult as Spenser strongly describes it to have been in his time. But this I am bound to say (irrespectively of the personal duties of Irish proprietors to their properties) that the intercourse of Englishmen with Ireland ought not to be limited, as it now mainly is, to regimental officers fretted by the tedium of provincial barracks, and an occasional tourist, or angler for salmon at Ballyshannon. The feeling of being neglected is one among the more reasonable causes of existing discontent, and of this alone I mean here to speak. Every Englishman who in a genial spirit travels or abides in

Ireland—and the demand does not go beyond common courtesy—is rendering service to both countries.

I write this soon after one of the abortive Fenian outbreaks—a mad and impotent insurrection, the seeds of which were sown on other soil than that of Ireland. I have seen enough of the Irish population of the great cities in the United States, to know how dangerous an element this has become by numbers and organisation—not so much to England as to the country which has received and given too early citizenship to this migrating multitude. The Irish population of New York, armed with this citizenship, becomes a fertile source of political dishonesty and international wrong. It is one among the several hindrances to the salutary working of the American Constitution, and will probably concur with other causes in compelling certain changes, expedient if not necessary, for the future welfare of that great nation.

The alteration in the general aspect and actual state of Ireland, since I first knew the country sixty years ago, is very striking. The ameliorations attained, despite famine, Fenianism, agrarian disturbances, and religious hatreds, are such in amount as to give good augury for the future, even should legislation do little more than it has hitherto done to assist and direct the natural resources of the country. If the Land question can be settled on sound principles, and ready practical application, much will be done towards this happier future. Geology forbids any expectation of it, but a six-foot bed of coal, stretching over the area of a midland Irish county, would be the best collateral aid to legislation for Ireland.

I graduated at Edinburgh in the autumn of 1811. Two friends with whom I was closely associated in preparing for the examination, Professor Alison and Dr. Gregory, are long since dead. The eminence of the former as a physiologist is well known ; and his amiable private qualities are still fresh in the memory of his friends. I took as the subject of my Latin thesis in graduation the ' Diseases of Iceland ; ' a subject I had studied with some interest during the four months I passed in that island. I dedicated it to my friend Geir Vidalin, the Bishop of Iceland at that time. With this simple-hearted and excellent man I had much pleasant intercourse at Rejkiavik—a great relief, especially at the moment when anxiously awaiting the arrival of the vessel that was to convey us back to England. My intercourse with Bishop Vidalin was carried on almost wholly in Latin. What spot other than Iceland could have afforded the picture of a Bishop, coming home to a small and rude timber-house from his day of sea-fishing in the Faxe-Fiord, and sitting down to Latin conversation with an English stranger! If his Latinity did not reach the level of Erasmus's ' Colloquies,' it certainly was better than any I could reciprocate with him ; impeded especially as I was by that perverse fashion of English pronunciation, which even Edinburgh teaching had only partially removed.

At the time of taking my degree, three years were

yet wanting of the age required for admission to the College of Physicians in London ; and looking to this place as my future destination, I formed my plans accordingly. Of the interval thus left at my disposal I appropriated the first part to a scheme of travel, not very closely defined, but embracing generally as much of the Mediterranean, and the countries bordering on it, as might be possible at this strange and eventful time of European history. I felt solicitous to accomplish all I could at an early period of life ; not then venturing to presume on the facilities for travel I afterwards obtained, and have so freely used.

Of this eastern voyage, I may here give a cursory sketch, justified in this exception to the rest of my narrative by the condition of Europe just noticed, and by the strange contrasts between travelling as it then was, and what it has become at the present day.

CHAPTER IV.

EARLY in 1812 I quitted England on this Mediterranean voyage—a period when Napoleon was about to pour upon Russia the armies of France, Italy, and Germany ; while in the Peninsula the Duke of Wellington was preparing the campaign which won the battle of Salamanca and carried the English army to Madrid. To the wars which thus shook Europe was added that unhappy one of more recent origin between England and the United States—a war chiefly of privateers on this side the Atlantic ; but not on that account indifferent to the English traveller, whose route in these days lay chiefly on the seas. This is one of the special brutalities of warfare which civilization, if really progressive as we deem it, is bound effectively to abolish.

Seeking to combine professional with other objects, I made Portugal my first landing point ; and though wholly unconnected with the army, spent much of my three months' stay in that country in diligent attendance on the Military Hospitals at Santarem, Abrantes, Niza, &c. The storming of Badajoz had been one of the most recent events of the war ; and the Convents at these several places appropriated as hospitals, were crowded to the utmost with the wounded and sick—

the wounds brought in from this desperate assault of Badajoz being singularly severe in kind. Everywhere I saw proofs of the watchful care the Duke of Wellington exercised over the medical branches of the service, even when himself most actively engaged elsewhere—a remark which indeed might equally apply to every other department connected with the army he commanded. He had, as is well known, an eye which kept strict watch over all; and a strong will, based on quick and upright judgment, to control abuses wherever they appeared. Though twice in the Peninsula during the war, and at momentous periods, it never happened to me to meet him there. But everywhere I witnessed the wonderful influence of his name and authority, even in those portions of the army furthest removed from his presence. I happened to be dining with Sir Charles Stuart (Lord Stuart de Rothesay) and another member of the Regency at Lisbon, in July, when Lord Clinton, charged with the Duke's despatches, rushed into the dinner-room, bringing the first tidings of the battle and victory of Salamanca, and asking a vessel for immediate passage to England. The interruption was in every sense a welcome one, and cordially hailed as such.

While gaining various good from the military hospital practice I witnessed in Portugal, I gave all medical aid in my power to the Hospital officers laboriously employed there; seeking to make this some compensation for the advantage of being myself ranked and provided for as a Major on the Commissariat list. Without such privilege indeed as to provisions and quarters, travelling through the country at this time would have been difficult, if not impossible. Receiving daily rations for myself, my servant and horse, and billeted on private houses on my route, this became the nearest approach I have ever made to the actual life of a soldier. I think I may say that I was not a harsh tenant of the quarters allotted to me in these private dwellings; and it happened in two or three instances that I came into the most friendly relations with the Portuguese families—some of them belonging to the higher classes—upon whom I was thus unceremoniously intruded. My residence at Santarem was more especially agreeable to me in this way, from bringing me into the best family society the place then afforded.

During my stay in this country I wrote a paper on the 'Volcanic Rocks of Iceland,' for the Lisbon Academy of Sciences; which, translated by Senhor Andrada, one of its members, was read before the Academy, and printed, I believe, in their Transactions. This led to my being elected a member of the Academy—my earliest honour of this kind.

Leaving Portugal, I proceeded by Gibraltar, Majorca, and Sardinia to Sicily, visiting the most interesting points in this island—then, as ever, the pride of the Mediterranean Sea. I ascended Etna exactly two years after I had been on the summit of Hecla; and passed a week in the Lipari Isles—a volcanic group much too rarely visited, seeing the singular variety of its volcanic products and all besides that it offers to the naturalist. Obsidian rocks, which in Iceland I had made a long

H

and arduous journey to see, are here brought massively before the eye, as in the castle-rock of Lipari; or curiously commingled, by community of origin, with the vast pumice beds spread over different parts of the island. Here too I discovered the Boracic acid *in situ*, at the bottom of the great crater of the Isle of Volcano; specimens of which had before been seen and described by Dolomieu, but without any knowledge of their exact locality.

At Palermo (then garrisoned by English troops, and governed in effect by Lord William Bentinck), I became intimate with Piazzi, well known as the discoverer of Ceres. This body stands first in date of that strange series of erratic planetoids, between Mars and Jupiter; so long limited to four in number, now counted up to more than a hundred, and multiplying every year under the keen eye of modern astronomy, to the discomfiture of those who sought only in the heathen mythology for the needful nomenclature. Piazzi's original discovery has the stronger historical mark set upon it from the fact of its having been made on the first night of the nineteenth century,—a century which, though yet only two-thirds completed, already comprises within itself many entire ages of human progress. The intellectual measurement of time differs greatly from that of history.

During my stay at Palermo I attended the debates in the Chambers of the Sicilian Parliament—an unavailing attempt, almost ludicrous in its details, to plant the English Constitution on a soil wholly unfitted for its reception. I came away from these Assemblies with a thorough conviction of what would be their speedy fate. They collapsed on the departure of the English troops, and the restoration of that effete monarchy destined to rule half a century longer over this fair part of Italy.*

I may note as an index of times gone by, though still recent for such a spectacle, that, in the voyage from Gibraltar to Sicily, I twice encountered an Algerine pirate squadron; and on the second occasion witnessed some of the violent outrages they committed on the southern coast of Sardinia. Yet at this time the naval power of England was supreme on the Mediterranean Sea! A few years later we redeemed ourselves from this merited reproach. In the spring of 1815 I saw, in the port of Genoa, the magnificent fleet with which Lord Exmouth the following year brought these outrages to an end.

From Sicily I proceeded to Zante and others of the Ionian Isles then in our possession; and in the succeeding six months travelled over various parts of Albania, Thessaly, Macedonia, and the more classical parts of Greece. The narrative of these travels was published in 1815, and went through two editions. This work, however, was impaired as to its completeness by the loss, or rather robbery, in Albania of a large

* In one of his admirable despatches from Vienna, the Duke of Wellington relates a conversation with the Emperor of Russia in which he quoted the utter failure of the constitution given to Sicily, as a caution against ever interfering, save in cases of absolute necessity, with the internal concerns of other countries. Liberal institutions, however sound in principle, are valueless as a gift, unless you have men fitted to administer them. Sicily had none such; and they cannot be suddenly created.

part of my papers, an incident to which I have elsewhere alluded—very mortifying at the time, but soon
forgotten, as things much more important are, in the
rapid passages of life.

Though the name of English physician brought many
patients to me in Turkey, of all races and ranks—Turks,
Greeks, and Albanians—I cannot speak of any gain of
professional knowledge from this part of my travels. I
have already alluded to the strange and insalutary
practice almost forced upon a physician by the ignorance
and vices of Turkish rulers and their subordinates. It
is a tax paid for the name of Hakim, and certain
facilities and privileges, hardly worth the price. Two
visits to Janina, the capital at that time of Ali Pasha's
large dominion, and two also to Larissa, in Thessaly,
the residence of his son Veli Pasha, showed me much of
this semi-barbarous farce of physic—somewhat amusing
for a time, worse than wearisome in its repetition.

An almost daily summons to his Palace during my
residence at Janina taught me thoroughly the character
of Ali Pasha—the mixture of strength, ferocity, and
cunning which had rendered him absolute over two
millions of subjects, and some of the fairest parts of
Greece—the superstition and sensuality which enslaved
him to himself. My visits to him made me also casually
the witness of many strange scenes of treachery and
bloodshed—strikingly indicative of the man, and a
cause of constant terror to all around him, and especially
to the Greek population living under his rule. Some of
these I have related in my ' Travels ;' but others I then

refrained from mentioning ; knowing that what I published would reach him in some shape or other, and that
certain persons still about him might be compromised
by the narrative.   It was his policy at this time to court
connection with England ; and this, with a certain show
of gratitude for my medical services to him, gave me
unwonted facilities in travelling through unfrequented or
dangerous parts of the country.   He stole indeed, as
elsewhere related, some of the fruits of my travel, and
put various hindrances in the way of my finally leaving
Janina ; but personal apprehension I never felt, though
for two months quite alone in my several Albanian
journeys.*

On two occasions, indeed, I was exposed to a sudden
burst of anger, speedily smothered by the consummate
cunning of the man.   A conversation on poisons,

---

* Two interviews with Meheńiet Ali, when I was first in Egypt, gave
me some means of comparing these two remarkable men, alike in origin
and fortune.   Both had handsome features, expressing strong natural
intellect and stronger will ; but there was a lurking devilry and cunning
even in the happiest moods of Ali Pasha's face, which contrasted un-
favourably with the more *civilised* countenance of Mehemet Ali.   Lord
Byron, as his poetry at least tells us, did not see this in the former ; but
his single interview could not well compare with my long and various
intercourse.   The *metrical necessities* of a poet (even about rhyme, as Butler
says in a happy couplet) are often recognised in the distortion or colouring of facts.   A curious instance of this occurs in two lines of Byron's
description of Tepeleni, the place where he had his interview with Ali
Pasha, and which I twice visited three years later :—

> ' The sun had sunk behind vast Tomarit,
>   And Laos, wide and fierce, came roaring by.'

Now, the great mountain Tomarit (the ancient Mons Tomarus) lies about
thirty miles *north-east* of Tepeleni ; and Laos I suspect to be a poetical
substitution for Aous, a name difficult to embody in verse.

designedly but warily brought on, ended by his asking me whether I knew of any poison which, put on the mouthpiece of a pipe, or given in coffee, might slowly and silently kill, leaving no note behind. The instant and short answer I gave that, 'as a physician I had studied how to save life, not to destroy it,' was probably, as I judged from his face, faithfully translated to him. He quitted the subject abruptly, and never afterwards reverted to it.

The other occasion was one that curiously showed the activity and astuteness of his government. He one day sent for me to his palace, and after more than that wonted prelude of affection which was one of his arts, put into my hands an English written paper, which he entreated me to translate to him, his English interpreter being then absent from Janina. Casting my eye over the first few lines, and then looking at the signature, I saw that it was a despatch from Sir R. Liston, our Ambassador at Constantinople, to Lord Castlereagh— probably connected with those important relations to the Porte at this particular time, in which Ali Pasha had a direct interest of his own. Putting the despatch at once aside, I stated through the Dragoman who stood awaiting my Italian translation of it, that this was a paper I ought neither to read myself or translate to others. My refusal seemingly amazed the Dragoman as well as his master; and under a somewhat vehement dictation of the Pasha, I was again pressed to assent. My persistent refusal evidently angered him much, and my visit came abruptly to an end. But the next day he received me with his wonted show of cordiality, and without any reference to what had passed between us. Mr. Foresti, our minister, was not at Janina at this time ; but I learnt from him afterwards some curious particulars as to the manner in which, by connivance with couriers, despatches (not English alone) were frequently intercepted, examined, and then resealed and forwarded to their destination.

Two visits to Veli Pasha, representing his father Ali Pasha in Thessaly, showed me another aspect of this Turco-Albanian sovereignty, modified by the subordinate position and milder character of the man. But these journeys were far more interesting in making me familiar with that grand region of Thessaly which blends itself in every part with Grecian history and mythology from the earliest ages. The names of Pindus, Olympus, Ossa and Pelion—of the Peneus, Tempe and Pieria—might alone invite travellers to a country, now rarely visited, simply because out of the direct reach of steamers and locomotives. These new modes of motion, while they extend linear distances of travel, narrow the view of all that lies outside their hard undeviating lines. Something has been gained, but much has been lost to the instruction as well as to the poetry of travel, by the new facilities given to it.

I have mentioned elsewhere my fondness for river scenery. My journeys in Thessaly enabled me to follow the course of the Peneus without interruption, from its sources in Pindus to its issue in the Ægean Sea—a route of infinite interest throughout, as well from classical association as from the various grandeur of its scenery. Olympus, Pindus, Ossa, Pelion, and Othrys all enter at different points into the mountain portion of the landscape. The 'Ιθώμη κλωμακόεσσα of Homer, represented to the traveller by the wonderful rocks of Meteora, forms the first great feature in the valley after the Peneus has emerged from its mountain recesses. The vale, or rather ravine, of Tempe is the last before it reaches the sea. Homeric names and sites, as well as others of Grecian history and mythology, are scattered everywhere over this region, carrying the mind back to times when truth and fiction are so mingled together that history itself runs into poetry as the fairest inter- preter. In the first volume of my 'Travels,' I have given what I think ample evidence, from Strabo, Livy, Eustathius, &c., of the identity of the Meteora Rocks with the Ithome of Homer.* The Monasteries, still eight or nine in number, isolated from the world on their several summits, were visited by Biornstahl a century ago, and are vividly described by Mr. Curzon in his 'Monasteries of the Levant.' I might almost have noted among my perils of travel, the ascent I made to one of these Monasteries—enclosed in a net, and swing- ing in open air for some minutes, while reaching the perpendicular height, as I conjecture, of about 180 feet ; and then finding, under a wooden shed, and working at a decayed windlass, three or four old and decrepit monks

---

* They are probably denoted at later date by the appropriate name of Gomphos or Gomphi—the scene of Cæsar's first success after crossing the chain of Pindus; a success sternly used.

to whom I had been indebted for the ascent, and by whom I was to be let down in like aerial way. No accident occurred, but neither was there any discovery of manuscripts to reward the adventure. All that I could see of this kind was worthless.

Coming from Thessaly to Delphi by the somewhat unwonted route of Mount Œta and the Tetrapolis of Doris—thence to Livadia and Thebes, and across the ridge of Cithæron then deeply covered with snow, I reached Athens on the first day of January, 1813. The month I passed there is strongly impressed on my memory. It was during the Turkish rule; and of the mere town of Athens, as it then was, scarcely a vestige remained, when I visited it with my friend the Dean of Westminster, forty-eight years afterwards. I have sought, as far as memory served me, to compare the impressions made on my mind at the two periods, thus distant, by that grand scenery of nature and those wonderful works of art which made Athens the 'eye of Greece,' at a time when Greece was the eye of the known world. Such comparison, whatever its reality, has its chief value to me as a test of my own feelings. All I can venture to affirm is, that time has not yet dimmed my sense as applied to these objects. I even believe that my enjoyment of them has been augmented and matured by the teachings of intermediate life.

I have a pleasant remembrance also of this month in Athens, from the society collected there at that time— Keppel Craven, Sir W. Gell, and Mr. Gandy, on their mission from the Dilettanti Society; Mr. North (afterwards Lord Guilford); Cockerell, Gropius, Haller, Lusieri, &c. We lived intimately together, while lodged in the houses of different Greek families of the place. I myself lived in the next house to that of Lord Byron's 'Maid of Athens,' and saw her and her sisters familiarly every day. Her youthful beauty, though somewhat embellished by the warmth of poetry, was such as might well attract the fancy of the poet. I found this a much more genial fashion of life than is afforded by the hotels of modern Athens, which, within sight of the Temples of Minerva and Theseus, mimic in miniature all that is most familiar in those of Western Europe. I am forced further to avow my feeling that the town in decay, under Turkish rule, harmonised better with the memories of ancient Athens—or, at least, intruded less upon them—than does the modern City; a feeble copy of a third-rate European capital, and utterly discordant in its associations with all around it. The pedantic adaptation of classical names to these creations of the day suggests nothing but a disagreeable feeling of incongruity. It would be well, indeed, if such incongruity were the sole or worst flaw in the feeble fabric of the Kingdom of Greece.

My journey through Argolis and other parts of the Morea was greatly impeded by the unwonted severity of the season. It was, in fact, the very winter which destroyed the French army retreating from Moscow, and spread its severity over all Europe. The valleys and plains of Arcadia, as well as its mountains, were deeply covered with snow for several weeks ; and more than once I was forced to retrace my route from losing all road or track beyond. It was strange to see the Citadel of Argos, the grand ruins of Mycenæ, and the sites of the Isthmian and Nemean Games thus covered ; and the solitary columns left at Nemea rising from amidst a waste of snow.*

As my travels in Turkey have been published, I will not linger further on these stray recollections of my first Eastern travel. I occupied four months in returning to England, three of which were passed in traversing Spain from Alicante through Madrid to Bilbao—a journey of some difficulty, as the French had still only partially evacuated the country, and the marks of years of war were everywhere deeply branded on its face ; more deeply from the irregular form this warfare had recently assumed. I have mentioned elsewhere my narrow escape of being taken prisoner by Harispe's cavalry near Castalla. It was the last movement of Suchet's army in the beautiful province of Valencia. I had gone to Castalla, to visit the Pantana, the magnificent artificial reservoir for irrigation, in the vicinity of that town ;—a silent reproach of a past century to the present age of Spanish sovereignty.

I had a most agreeable fellow-traveller, during this Spanish journey, in Frederick Lord Guilford ; who, to the humour and admirable temper hereditary in the North family, added much various but very eccentric

---

* My travels led me also to the scene of the Pythian and Olympic Games, ennobled by the finest Lyric poetry of Greece. The latter site, which I visited in a separate excursion from Zante, might possibly, notwithstanding the spoliation by Roman conquerors, still yield something to research.

learning of his own.* A fair scholar, he nevertheless revelled more in the loose and profligate literature of the Byzantine times than in that of the older classics. Becoming afterwards Chancellor of the University of Corfu, he prided himself as much on his addresses in the Romaic Greek of the Ionian Isles, as he could have done if speaking the purest Ionic of the classical ages. Our first intimacy at Athens was renewed at Zante ; and from thence we travelled together to England, parting only under the chestnut trees of Bushy Park. I still picture him in my travelling recollections, as he stood, habited in the Windsor uniform of that day, over the excavations he was making near the Lantern of Demosthenes at Athens ; or as in Spain he used patiently to sit on his camp-stool under a cork tree, reading the Δειπνοσοφισταὶ of Athenæus, while our carriage mules were feeding, or any accident detained us. It was a

---

* It was of the copious library of this Lord Guilford that his Sister, Lady C. Lindsay, used to say, and not without some justification, ' Frederick's library contains but two sorts of books—books that *cannot* be read, and books that *ought not* to be read.' I know only one person to whom I could now appeal for recollection of the dinners at his house in St. James's Place ; strangely heterogeneous in the guests, English and Foreign, but always genial and amusing. Of the six children of the Minister Lord North (three of them successively Earls of Guilford), I lived in intimate friendship with five to the time of their death. They had all, though under very different circumstances, the same happy temperament, and a wit which played gently over the surface of things, without personal offence. Four, if not five, of them died from the same cause, disease of the heart. Very few are now left to remember this generation of the family, of whom Lady Charlotte, perhaps the most agreeable, was the last survivor. Her playful letters were wrongfully obtained, and wrongfully used in the Queen's trial in 1821. The North papers coming to her by succession, have been variously brought into contemporary history.

loitering journey of weeks, and in this well suited his temperament both of body and mind.

A fortnight at Madrid showed us some curious spectacles consequent on the recent flight of King Joseph and his Court, and the retreat of the French army. At the theatres, bull-fights, and in the streets, the popular enthusiasm was strongly testified. Our party here, augmented by the arrival of two English noblemen, was everywhere warmly received. Free admission was given us to the theatres, both before and behind the scenes; and in the case of the Company of the Teatro de la Cruz, this familiarity was carried further by a reciprocal exchange of dinners, at which the merriment of songs and speech found very free licence. The Arsenias and Florimondas of the Company were present at these festivities, and testified by their demeanour that Le Sage's portraits had not been drawn for one age only. At this time of popular emotion the old dramas of Lope di Vega and Calderon were flung aside, and patriotic farces substituted, in which the Prosopopeia was often curiously used. I recollect one piece, in which not only England and Spain were personified, but also each separate province of Spain was thus represented, with the fitting varieties of dress and dialect.

At Madrid we heard of the great victory of Vittoria, and a fortnight afterwards were on the battle-field there, still bearing many marks of the fight, and of the flight that followed. The 149 cannon taken from King Joseph's army were still on the spot; and I gathered up, from

amidst broken carriages and other wrecks of war, many
manuscript papers, curiously illustrating the disordered
and discontented state of the French army at that time ;
but also showing that some of their officers had been
living in very amicable relations with Spanish ladies.
Here, too, and subsequently at Bilboa, I occupied myself in the military hospitals—crowded at Vittoria, not
only by the wounded in the battle there, but by the
numbers brought in from the three days' mountain
battles of the Pyrenees—the hardest and most bloody
struggle of the war. I witnessed their arrival, together
with the 2,500 prisoners taken in these fights. No spectacle more painful than that of the carriage of the
wounded, sick, and dying, in the midst of a campaign !
I have since seen it in Algeria, and on a much larger
scale in Virginia, during the late American struggle ;
but there mitigated as far as was possible by the excellent hospital provisions of the Federal army, which I
have never seen equalled elsewhere. Still it is in every
case the blackest page of war. The strategy, exploits,
and triumphs of the battle-field are all dimmed in looking at this inevitable sequel. It is needful to have
seen to comprehend it, for official despatches and history tell but little of the reality.

Our voyage to England, made in company with a
large fleet of transports conveying more than 2,000
French prisoners, told another part of the same sad
story. A long and rude passage across the Bay of Bis-
cay, and the fear of the prisoners rising on the feeble
crews of the transports, compelled precautions which

added much to the sufferings of these poor soldiers—
many of them conscripts newly and forcibly dragged to
the war—a sacrifice to the selfish and unsated ambition
of a single man.

Two years still remained to me before reaching the
age required by the College of Physicians. The earlier
part of this time I passed in London, pursuing medical
studies, while also enjoying a very desirable society, to
which the repute of having travelled in Iceland and
Greece mainly contributed. It was at this time that
the intimacy, ripening afterwards into friendship, was
formed with Lord Lansdowne, Lord Aberdeen, and Lord
Holland, which continued unbroken to the death of these
three eminent men. The tables at Lansdowne House
and Holland House were then, as they long continued
to be, an introduction to all that was most remarkable
in London society. At these dinners it was my good
fortune to be a frequent guest. During this period also
I saw much of Lord Byron, then in the fulness of his
fame; of Horner, Mackintosh, Sir Samuel Romilly,
Ward (Lord Dudley), Rogers, Sir Humphry Davy, the
Misses Berry, and another very conspicuous lady, to
whom the London world paid large homage in the
winter of 1814. This was Madame de Staël; a woman
sufficiently remarkable in her own qualities, intellectual
and social; invested at this time with the fame of a
political exile ; and bringing with her various fashions—
reminiscences to a few, novelties to the many—of that
Continental life from which Englishmen had so long

been separated. I first met her at a great dinner at Bridgewater House; whence the party adjourned in the evening to the opening of the British Gallery, of which our host the Marquis of Stafford was then President. The accident of her taking my arm during our stay in the crowded Gallery made me a witness of the curious eagerness to see and hear her which prevailed at the time. It also brought me immediately several invitations to meet her in society, from persons whom I had not known before. These things are characteristic, it must be owned, of what may be called foibles, as well as features, of London life. Time has done little since to alter them.

I saw much afterwards of Madame de Staël at her own house in Argyll Street, in those literary and political circles which she gathered round her, and where she declaimed or argued with all who could meet her with her own weapons and in her own language. Sir J. Mackintosh was the most frequent and expert of these intellectual combatants: and it was the combat most congenial to his own tastes. In some points there was a certain intellectual likeness between them; such as the power of putting an argument into its most pithy shape—what may be called a *wit of speech*, apart from that gift of *humour*, to which neither of them could lay much claim. Frequently too I used to sit alone with Madame de Staël at her fireside, to which she clung closely in the wintry cold of the spring of 1814. Her conversation, always earnest and eloquent, often fell upon my recent travels in the East. She had formed at this time the scheme of a work on the Crusades, fashioned upon the plan of Fénelon's 'Télémaque.' The outline of this she put in detail before me, seeking for such suggestions as I might be able to offer. I was obliged to confess my inability to render any aid worth having; explaining to her, what she did not sufficiently understand, that an intimacy with Turks and Turkish Pashas of the present day, such as mine was, would furnish few hints for the picture of Saladin, or of the Seljuk chiefs and warriors of that more romantic age. Her scheme never ripened into any reality.

One of the latest occasions of my meeting Madame de Staël was at a dinner at Sir Samuel Romilly's; well marked in my memory by the intelligence being received, while we were yet at table, of the entry of the Allied Armies into Paris. Her emotion was great, and ardently expressed, though leaving it somewhat doubtful whether pleasure or pain predominated. Her life had borne this mingled character throughout. In a single sentence she thus denotes her mental temperament—'Calme et animée; ce qu'il faut être, et ce que je ne suis pas.' Another trait she discloses, speaking of *les revenans*: 'Je n'y crois pas, mais je les crains.' She measured herself well in these self-avowals, to which another trait, less avowed, might perhaps have been added. From my own observation, as well as that of others, I was led to believe that she would willingly have surrendered something of her intellectual fame for a little more of personal beauty. She was ever curiously demonstrative of her arms, as the feature which best

I

satisfied this aspiration. A slip of paper often in her hand, and sedulously twisted during her eager conversation, might be a casual trick of habit, though there were some who gave it a more malicious interpretation. Even admitting this, however, and other foibles, Madame de Staël cannot be otherwise described than as a woman of extraordinary endowments.

Somewhat later in this year a proposal was made to me, through my Athens' friends, Keppel Craven and Sir W. Gell, attached as Chamberlains to the Princess of Wales, to attend upon Her Royal Highness as physician during the first year of her intended residence on the Continent. In forming this engagement for the short period still open to me, I was obliged to consider its bearing upon my future professional career. The decision to which I came I had no subsequent cause to regret. Irrespectively of the pleasure of passing this interval in Italy—a country for nearly twenty years shut out from English travel—I acquired many new friendships, valuable to me in every way in after-life. At this period, while Napoleon was still at Elba, the aspect of Europe clouded and unsettled throughout, and steam as a locomotive power yet unknown, the English travellers who reached Florence, Rome, and Naples were comparatively few in number, but somewhat more select in quality than those who now everywhere crowd Continental hotels. My previous intimacy with many of these families, and the position in which I myself travelled, gave me various advantages I could not otherwise have enjoyed. These circumstances, and still more the singular condition of

Europe at this time, just emerging from a stern military despotism, but with the despot still close at hand in his island-ambush, may warrant a slight fragmentary record of the journey for which I was thus engaged ; omitting various details of Courts, public receptions, and spectacles, which I find in my journal, but am not tempted to transcribe. I have never indeed been a practised relater of anecdotes ; and do not pretend, thus late in life, to take up the character.

To this narrative then, in its chief incidents, as to that of my earlier Mediterranean voyage, I give a short separate chapter. Of my subsequent annual journeys, much shorter as to time, and made when the world was in a more settled state (if such phrase be ever applicable to worldly affairs), I have already spoken generally ; and shall not need, unless incidentally, to revert to them again.

CHAPTER V.

LANDING at Hamburg from the Jason frigate, which
had been commissioned to the service of the Princess, we
found the place occupied by a swarm of Cossacks,
strangely contrasting with the other aspects of a commercial city; yet the contrast was hardly greater than
between Hamburg of that time—the mediæval Hanse
Town—with the City as it is now seen, one of the
handsomest as well as most prosperous in Europe.
I have visited it very often during the interval—once
directly after that great fire which swept away much of
the picturesque old Hamburg to make place for the more
formal architecture of the new. The other Hanse
Towns—Lubeck, Dantzig, Bremen, &c.—have undergone similar change since I first visited these curious
cities—the commercial creation of a period when the
rest of Europe was clouded by feudal darkness and
disorders.

The journey of ninety miles from Hamburg to Brunswick, aided by all the appliances that could be given,
marks in another way the changes that time has since
effected. It was then a toilsome travel of two days over
heavy sands, or through marshy thickets, on roads so

rudely fashioned that one of the Princess's carriages was upset even within sight of Brunswick. It is now an easy railroad journey of four or five hours.

We remained a fortnight in this quaint and solitary City, living in the Ducal palace—the last guests received there before those events of the next year, in which the life of the Duke came to an end. I saw and conversed much with him during our stay at Brunswick. His character was one strongly contrasted with that of his Sister, and each manifestly felt the disparity, though showing their consciousness of it in very different ways. There was a grave simplicity about the Duke, tinged with a shade of melancholy, which might almost by a superstitious observer have been interpreted as a fore-boding of evil at hand. He was in every sense superior to the formal little Court around him—a Court, I must admit, a good deal disturbed in its grave decorum by the sudden arrival of the Princess and her large suite, still under the joyousness of early travel, and not altogether mindful of the wonted proprieties of the place. Some of these breaches of decorum might almost be regarded as a retaliation on the part of the Princess for those dull formalities of the Brunswick palace in her youth, of which Lord Malmesbury has left so curious a narrative.

The halt of a day at Göttingen enabled me to visit the veteran Blumenbach, and to spend some time with him in his museum. At that time his collection of Crania was the most complete in Europe; and his de-ductions from them, however modified by later research, have in effect given basis to Craniology as a science; a fact admitted to me by Retzius, when I visited his more magnificent collection at Stockholm forty-four years afterwards. My visit to Blumenbach, hurried though it was, showed me the energy and clearness of his mind, little impaired by years. He had the happiness, among the greatest a man can have, of a definite object of pursuit, unlimited in its scope, and of deep interest in its conclusions. Blumenbach was not a phrenologist in the later sense of the term ; but he saw the ethnological value of those distinctions which only large and well-classified collections of crania can afford.

During a short stay at Cassel, the Princess was entertained at Wilhelmshöhe by the Elector, who came thither with his family to receive her. My love of volcanic rocks gave me interest in the groups of basaltic columns emerging above ground in these beautiful gardens, and furnishing picturesque material for their waterfalls and fountains. How strange and stormy that flow of human events which brought a second Napoleon to Wilhelmshöhe, stripped of his empire, and a prisoner of war !

At Strasburg, where we stayed some days, I saw much of Marshal Kellerman, Duc de Valmy, now more than eighty—a name and age bringing into memory the first battle and victory of the French Revolution. His reception of the Princess, whether under orders or not, was marked by more than ordinary attentions. These included a review, at which he commanded, of more than 8,000 troops—a great dinner, at which all the civil and military authorities were present—a ball, and a public night at the theatre. There was a strangeness about this demon-

stration, when remembering the fact that it was the
Duke of Brunswick, the father of the Princess, whom
Marshal Kellerman defeated at Valmy, in 1792. The
Marshal, as I knew, had this fully in his recollection.   I
have some doubts whether the Princess equally recognised it.   Her knowledge of the events amidst which
she had lived, as well as of their antecedents, was
curiously vague and inconsecutive; and the quick succession of places and persons in travelling did not amend
this deficiency.

From General Humbert and the staff officers of the
garrison of Strasburg we, as the suite of the Princess,
received many private civilities. In society with them it
was impossible not to note the ambiguous reserve with
which they spoke equally of the past and the future—a
sort of sullen restlessness, betokening beforehand the
events of the following year.   Defection from the Bour-
bon flag, if opportunity offered, was obvious, even to a
foreign and casual observer like myself. It was a strange
contrast to pass at once from this angry and distempered
military society to the quiet and recluse library of
Schweighauser, the learned editor of Polybius, Athenæus, and subsequently of Herodotus. On this last
work he was then actively engaged ; and I passed a
good deal of time with him, giving what aid I could
to his notes on the old Greek historian, from my
local knowledge of Marathon, Thermopylæ, and Platæa.
Men occupied like Schweighauser are to be envied,
even when their labours fall upon a careless or forgetful
world.

I had another interest at Strasburg, in the acquaintance I made there with Talma, the great tragic actor of his time. On one evening, after seeing him in his favourite character of Manlius Capitolinus, I supped and sat with him till after midnight. I never saw an actor of such striking demeanour on the stage. The figure and features of John Kemble were finer, but rigid and impassive compared with those of Talma. His birth and early life in England gave him intimate knowledge of our language ; and he recited with fervour some passages from Shakespeare, showing how well he understood and admired him. He told me (in reference to a comment I hazarded on his manner of recitation in Lafosse's tragedy) that, feeling painfully the monotonous mouthing of the French tragedians, it was his constant study, wherever the sense permitted, to disguise the rhyme by rapid enunciation or pauses, rather than put emphasis upon it. And of this he gave me at the moment some striking illustrations. Two or three times he spoke of Napoleon, whom he well knew personally ; but it was done with the reserve, so common at this period in France, rather repelling than inviting further conversation on the subject. I doubt not that he shared in the current belief that the career of the Emperor had not come to its end. But for this reserve I should gladly have questioned him as to the comments Napoleon is known to have made on his performance of certain characters on the stage. Anecdotes of this kind, and comments illustrative of the man who made them, indeed of every kind, lose so much of their reality by repetition, that it is well, where possible, to trace them back to their source.

Entering Switzerland by the unfrequented but very picturesque route of the Munster-Thal, our first halt was at Berne, where at this time were residing the Empress Maria Louisa and the Grand-Duchess Constantine. With these Imperial ladies, and especially the former, long visits were interchanged. On one of these evenings the Empress sang some Italian and German songs, accompanied by Count Neuperg, whose history became afterwards by marriage so closely associated with her own. One of these I recollect to have been Ferrari's beautiful air of ' L'Innamorata.' Maria Louisa's manner was quiet and pleasing, without any other marked character. Of the great captive then at Elba not a syllable, as far as I know, was uttered—a silence which told far more than any speech could have done. The remainder of her life gave full interpretation to it. All indeed that we have learnt of the elder Napoleon, even since his death, tells us how little his hard and selfish nature was fitted to awaken tender feelings in those with whom he lived.

A short stay at Geneva was singularly agreeable to me. I made the acquaintance there of many eminent men—Saussure, Sismondi, Pictet, Prévost, De la Rive, Decandolle, Maunoir, &c., and saw much of them either at their own houses or in more general society. It was a group of persons which might have given fame to a much larger city than Geneva. Political dissensions, the small scale of which never abates their bitterness, have done much since that time to disturb

this tranquil seat of science. Nor has there been wanting a certain admixture of that religious excitement,
for which, since the Reformation, Geneva has always
been signalised. Where the image of Calvin still stalks,
the opposite spirit is sure to be evoked.

I quitted the Princess here for a separate excursion
to Chamouni; rejoining her at Martigny, and thence
crossed into Italy by the Simplon. It was my first
passage over the Alps, since followed by many others
over the several Alpine passes—now, as well as the summits above them, become so familiar to English holiday
travel.* The adventures of Englishmen in climbing
these lofty summits, though of small profit to science,
are an index of national energy, which it would be wrong
to undervalue. But at the time of which I am speaking,
Switzerland, now so prolific of pleasure and enterprise,
was known to our youth but as a barren lesson of school
geography. At that date the conception of railroads
crossing the Alps or of tunnels cut underneath them,
would have been ranked among the vagaries of lunacy
or Laputan philosophy. It is needful to go back to
these prior times, to gain any due conception of the
gigantic strides science has made in controlling and
applying the natural elements which surround us.

It was pleasant to begin Italian life by two days on
the Isola Bella, the island-palace of the Conte Borromeo,

---

* An old London and Dover mail coach had been purchased for the
conveyance of some of the servants and baggage of the Princess. It was a
whimsical sight this coach offered when scaling the Simplon, with all the
old English designations still upon its panels. Arrived at Naples, King
Joachim admired and purchased it ; but his dethronement soon afterwards
ended also the career of the Dover mail in Italy.

who entertained us with a magnificent hospitality, both on his island and lake. The friendship I then formed with this excellent and accomplished family was pleasantly renewed in Italy many years afterwards, though now again broken by accumulated years of absence.

Ten days were passed at Milan amidst the novelties of an Italian society, including most of the principal titled families and officials of this city. I found leisure however for my own more particular pursuits ; passing much time in the Ambrosian Library, where I watched with great interest the operations of Angelo Mai (afterwards Cardinal) in deciphering the Palimpsest MSS. found in this celebrated library. Very recently he had discovered fragments of the Iliad, amounting to nearly 800 lines, inscribed on the back of some ancient drawings (uncertain in date) of scenes in the poem. He sent me at a later time, after his translation to Rome and the larger labours of the Vatican Library, the volume containing those portions of the ' *De Republicâ* ' of Cicero, which he had rescued from their palimpsestic obscurity. Even allowing for very imperfect restoration, it scarcely takes rank with Cicero's other treatises. Fragments of the lost books of Livy or Tacitus, or Sylla's Autobiography, or some of the missing works of Julius Cæsar, or an original play of Menander, would have been deemed by many a happier discovery.* There was something very prepossessing in the quiet

---

* I look forward with much interest to the chances of recovery, under the auspices of the present Government, of some of those literary treasures of antiquity which still lie buried underneath the Herculaneum tufa. It is

simplicity of Mai, and his entire devotion to the work in his hands—a lightsome labour to his mind. He honoured the grade of Cardinal more than he was honoured by it.

One of the Directors of the Ambrosian Library at this time was Amoretti, the author of a work 'Sulla Raddomanzia'—the *Scienza*, as he willingly termed it, of the Divining Rod. The whole mind of this good old man was engrossed with this one subject, and he sedulously sought to bring me over to his belief. The experiments he made before the Princess carried sources of fallacy on the very face of them ; but his gentle and earnest simplicity forbade any exposure of these self-deceptions. There are many cases in life where to convince, even of error, is a breach of the charity we owe to one another.

I spent more profitable time at Milan in the geological collections of Breislak and Brocchi, and in the observatory of Oriani. Science, like society, was breathing now more freely again, after the oppression of so many years of military rule. The hand of Napoleon, indeed, lay less heavy on what had some accordance with his own tastes, than upon literature and those other objects of human pursuit to which genius seeks to press its way. But the shade of despotism is broad as well as gloomy, and neither object nor distance can give exemption from its sinister influence.

one of the few chances left open for such recovery. Future excavations may possibly afford us papyri in more perfect preservation, or fragments of greater literary value than those obtained from the very limited research hitherto directed to this spot.

In the reception of the Princess at the miniature Court of Modena, I at once recognised the Duke and Duchess as the Archduke Francis and Princess Beatrice of Sardinia, whom I had seen at Cagliari two years before, in that forlorn refuge of royalty. Fifty years have since sufficed to raise what was then the meagre island-court of Sardinia to the Sovereignty of a Kingdom of Italy; abolishing Modena, with other more important States, in the act of change. The destiny of this new kingdom is one of the most interesting elements in the future history of Europe, irrespectively even of that futile and mischievous figment called ' the balance of power.' If held together in its integrity, the religious as well as the political relations of European States will inevitably undergo much change from the Italian unity thus established.

At Bologna I became acquainted with that marvellous master of languages, Mezzofanti, and was able to satisfy myself that his extraordinary faculty had not been exaggerated by common report. Looking at the special endowment of this man, one may well ask what portion of the brain gives lodgment to so wonderful a museum of words, and to their catenation in series of some thirty languages? Or, again, whence comes it that a faculty thus strange dominates so largely in some men (Pico di Mirandola, Crichton, Wotton, Mezzofanti, &c.), and is so deficient in others? Anatomy and Physiology render no answer, and are in truth entirely silent as to the strange mechanism of memory, whatever its objects and methods. Hypothesis indeed has been frequently at work here, as on other problems of kindred nature, but vainly as regards any intelligible results. I saw too little of Mezzofanti to justify me in applying to him the opinion that a singular excellence in one faculty involves defect in others—an opinion strikingly contradicted in the case of Lord Macaulay, whose wonderful memory served but as a substratum to his other faculties. I may merely say that I noticed no expression of intellect in Mezzofanti that would be thought remarkable. But my observation was much too short to be put on record to this effect.

A journey over the Apennines on a boisterous night was lightened by meeting at the mountainous village of Lojano, with Lord and Lady Holland and their family, arrested here by the storm. A homely supper, got up impromptu at midnight in a rude mountain hostelry, was well seasoned by its novelty, and by the various character and antecedents of the guests thus strangely brought together. This midnight meal in the Apennines was the first occasion in which the Princess of Wales and Lady Holland had come into actual intercourse. The entire diversity of the two personages gave little likelihood of its being afterwards renewed.

Amidst the more courtly festivities at Florence, there occurred one quiet evening visit to the Countess Albany—the remaining representative of the Pretender's family, but yet more closely associated with the name and fame of Alfieri. She retained, even at this time, a certain dignified charm of conversation and manner, explaining in part the incidents of her past romantic life, though leaving much to be assigned to the influence of other causes. There were some general allusions to these past events, but for obvious reasons they could not be pursued into detail. Madame d'Albany died nine years after this visit to her at Florence.

The week passed at Rome, on our way to Naples, might almost be called one of toil, such were the demands upon it. All the private time I could myself obtain was small compared with that in which my attendance was required with the Princess, in the various ceremonies, spectacles, and festivities of which she was the object. Though putting some hindrances in the way, I had no reason on the whole to complain of this requisition. It showed me easily and agreeably many things which in no other way I could have seen. Rome at this moment was crowded with personages known more or less—for better or for worse—in the history of the time. Many of these were expatriated Princes, and their followers in adversity ; awaiting the decision of the Congress of Vienna, and other incidents hanging over them.

The Pope, Pius VII., venerable from age, character, and misfortunes bravely borne, deservedly held first rank in the number. I was in attendance on the Princess when she visited him at his palace on Monte Cavallo. I twice saw him at High-Mass—the second time on the festival day of St. Carlo di Borromeo, when numerous Cardinals were present, and the celebration had much of magnificence. I still possess, and duly value, a rosary of blood-stones which this venerable Pontiff sent me the day before I left Rome. He had been recently restored to his temporal dominion, very soon to quit it again as a refugee.

The other personages here at this time were Charles IV. of Spain, his Queen, the Infante Don Paolo, and Godoy—the Queen of Etruria, a Princess of Sardinia, a Prince of Saxe-Gotha, Louis the ex-King of Holland, Lucien Bonaparte and his wife, the Princess Piombino, Cardinal Fesch, Prince Poniatowski, &c. In the daily intercourse with these several persons, there was much to interest and amuse me. The Spanish royal family, by far the strangest embodied in these Roman recollections, became somewhat intimately known to me. I was professionally consulted by the Queen and Godoy, names inauspiciously connected in the recent history of Spain. I retain strongly in memory the picture of the four personages of this Royal Spanish group, with whom I more than once passed an hour in their apartments—the old King, bulky in body, vacant in face and mind, placidly indolent in his whole demeanour—the Queen, a woman whose countenance, voice, and figure might easily in older days have condemned her as a witch—the Infante, an ill-fashioned youth, who laughed idiotically when his mother alluded to the wine-mark on his face—and Godoy (Prince of the Peace), the shadow of a handsome man; pleasing in manner and common conversation, but showing no other quality to justify the influence he so long retained in the government of Spain. I met the same Royal party, fugitives again, at Venice the following year. It was a group strangely depicting royalty in its most effete form, and telling the tale óf long misgovernment in a country deserving a better fate. Death has since disposed of them all.

We saw much of the members of the Bonaparte family then at Rome. They dined with Her Royal Highness, and gave entertainments to her in return. The palace of Lucien (Prince of Canino), rich in works of art, was open freely to all her suite. A ball and concert he gave to the Princess was magnificent in the assemblage of the Roman nobility there, including seven or eight Cardinals. Chance led me on this occasion to have a long conversation with Louis, the ex-King of Holland, who possessed a charm in that gentle simplicity of manner, which won for him the affections of his Dutch subjects, and in winning these cost him his crown. He talked to me unaffectedly on this subject, and equally so on others of political concern. In carrying my memory back to these things, I am led to compare and contrast them with the character and fortunes of his extraordinary Son—destined, after prolonged exile and imprisonment, to become for a time the most powerful arbiter in the affairs of Europe. I have on the table before me at this moment the second volume of the ' Histoire de Jules-César '—the very magnificent folio copy with which I had been honoured as a present from the Emperor, in sequel to the first volume before received from him.* It is a curious contrast of royal authorship, as concerns the

* I have before mentioned that an article I wrote for the *Quarterly Review* (republished in my volume of *Essays*), of which the life and character of Julius Cæsar formed the chief subject, led to my being favoured by the gift of these volumes.

K

father and son, to compare these two splendid volumes
with that placid little work 'Marie, ou les Hollandaises,'
in which King Louis gently pictures the people over
whom he was allowed a brief rule, suspended when
it interfered with the purposes of a sterner and more
ambitious will.

I saw a good deal of Cardinal Fesch at Rome, and
had various conversations with him. I find in my notes
the record of one argument on the celibacy of the clergy;
a thesis on which, according to my recollections, he sustained his side of the question with more ingenuity than
sincerity. He was a man evidently cloaking strong
qualities of mind and temper under his ecclesiastical
garb. At this moment especially it was very needful
for him to exercise a cautious forbearance in his relations
to those around him.

I felt it a singular privilege to visit the galleries of
the Vatican and Capitol under the guidance of Canova,
who attended upon the Princess while at Rome. The
advantage, however, would have been greater had there
been less of royalty and crowd on these several occasions. The objects of highest art, and the comments of
great artists upon them, can only be duly appreciated
when mind and body are at rest from other things. The
atmosphere of a crowd is always an unwholesome one,
mentally as well as physically.

We reached Naples early in November, King Joachim
meeting the Princess at Aversa, and bringing her to his
capital with much military show. Policy, or what at
this time was supposed such, blended itself here with

the love of pomp and display innate in his temperament. The four months we passed at Naples—the closing period of his reign—were coloured in every way by the personal character of the man. It was a time of continuous fête and revelry—of balls, masquerades, and operas—of levées, processions, and military reviews—of boar-hunts and fishing parties, and numerous other festivities by land and sea. In all these Murat himself was the conspicuous figure, and well pleased to be so. Tall and masculine in person ; his features well formed, but expressing little beyond good nature and a rude energy and consciousness of physical power ; his black hair flowing in curls over his shoulders; his hat gorgeous with plumes ; his whole dress carrying an air of masquerade —this was the general aspect of the man, well picturing the ardent chieftain of cavalry in Napoleon's great campaigns. Amidst the luxurious life of Naples, indeed, his feelings and conversation often reverted to the time when he was hotly engaged with Cossack bands on the plains of Poland and Russia. I have seen him dressed as a Cossack Chief at a court masquerade ; and parading the Strada di Toledo, with a long suite of his old companions in war, in similar costume. He was endowed with a large amount of pure animal vitality, which pleasurably expended itself in the active deeds of war but found no sufficient vent in peace, even when called upon to act the king. I think he was personally popular with his Neapolitan subjects, including the Lazzaroni, who had their peculiar way of describing with the fingers his gait on horseback, and the waving of his plumes.

With all his fantasies of dress, there was a jovial kindness of temperament, which made his presence agreeable to the public eye. I mention his popularity, however, with the distrust I always feel for the judgment of travellers on a matter of this kind, founded, as it generally is, on partial instances, often on the mere personal feelings of the narrator.

His Queen, the Sister of Napoleon, required and deserved more study. Under her fine and feminine features lay a depth of thought—at this time, as it seemed to me, verging upon melancholy. I doubt not, indeed, from what I saw and heard, that she was keenly sensible of the crisis then hanging over the fortunes of her family. Her qualities were very different, and loftier than those of her husband; and both I believe to have been fully conscious of this disparity. Many obvious causes rendered her less popular than him, both in the Palace and among the people. I had constant opportunities of observing them together in the various Court festivities, at all which she was present; though, as I could fancy, from obligation (or from jealousy, as some surmised) rather than real pleasure. Curiously enough, the English country dance, now almost lost to ourselves, was in high fashion at this time at Naples; and as my own days of youth were not yet gone by, it often happened to me at the Court balls to stand with Murat and his Queen in the same country dance—she much the most graceful dancer as well as most dignified personage of her Court.

One of these occasions is deeply marked in my

memory. It was a great ball given by Count Mosburg, the Minister of Finance, on one of the first days of March. All belonging to the Neapolitan Court were present ; the Princess of Wales and her suite ; the principal nobility of Naples and many foreigners. Among the latter was the Countess Walewski, very recently arrived from Elba with her young son ; and attracting much attention from her known relation to the great prisoner there, as well as from the graces of her own person and manner. Her sudden presence at Naples, and certain other collateral incidents, excited suspicions without defining them. It was that vague whisper which often precedes some event close at hand. The ball of which I am speaking afforded the solution in a sudden and startling way. Everything went on according to the wonted fashion of such festivities until about 11 o'clock—the King and Queen, with the principal persons of their Court, being at that moment engaged in the figures of an English country dance. Count Mosburg, our host, was suddenly summoned out of the room. He speedily returned, went up to the King, and whispered intelligence to him, which he instantly communicated in similar way to the Queen. They both disappeared from the dance, and the assembly itself was at once dissolved ; each guest carrying away some dim surmise of what had happened. The intelligence, in fact, was the escape of Napoleon from Elba—that romantic exploit which has already passed into history as one of the most extraordinary events of the age in which we live. His departure only was known at this time ; but I was still at Naples when the intelligence came of Napoleon's first successes in France.

Many English were present at this ball ; amongst whom I recollect the Duke of Bedford, Lord and Lady Holland, Lord and Lady Conyngham, Lord and Lady Oxford, Lord Gage, Lord Clare, &c. Of these only Lord Gage is now alive to recollect the scene.

Murat was resplendent on horseback, and felt himself to be so. He dwarfed all his numerous suite in person and fine horsemanship, and revelled in his superiority. Yet on one occasion, at a great boar-hunt in the country, I saw him thrown from an English blood-mare which he had mounted for the first time. A large and fierce boar rushed at him—the horse reared, and the King slipped off—his fall *sheltered*, and the boar repelled, by a crowd of equerries and other officers. This incident, as I was told, much annoyed him. I now and then accompanied his riding parties ; and on one occasion, at a review of the regiments of guards, rode close to him in a charge of cavalry on a square of infantry—his Queen placed within the square. It was curious to witness his elation and eagerness even in this petty mimicry of fight. The close of his career, both of royalty and life, came speedily in sequel to it.

Amongst the English visitors at Naples, parties were numerous to Pompeii, Vesuvius, Baia, and the other points around this beautiful bay—all fresh then to the English eye, and not yet overlaid with guide-books and guides. One of my several visits to Pompeii was made with Lord and Lady Holland and the Duke of Bedford ;

another with the Princess of Wales, Countess Walewski, M. Beaufremont, &c. Madame Walewski was accompanied by her son ; then a boy seven or eight years of age, since known to me as French Ambassador in London, and holding high positions under the second French Empire. More than once I have since talked to him about these events of his boyhood, and this visit to Pompeii as one of them. He aided me much by his letters of recommendation in my last visit to the Eastern province of Algeria. His likeness in feature to his presumed father, the first Napoleon, is well known. His death anteceded but a short time the events which have just hurried the Second Empire to its end.

On a later occasion I joined Lord and Lady Holland, Lord John Russell, and General Fox, in an excursion to Pæstum—a journey of four or five days it might rather be called, rendered such by the slow rate at which alone Lady Holland would consent to travel, either here or elsewhere. Two nights in going and returning were passed at the forest-palace of Persano, by invitation of the King. In this wild and secluded spot, devoted to the field-sports of Neapolitan princes, we found ample entertainment provided for us; and under these happy conditions of companionship in travel, and reception on the way, it was impossible to quarrel with the duration of the journey. The mere sight of these three temples of the ancient Posidonia, made more impressive by the solitude surrounding them, was an ample reward.

My fondness for volcanic scenery was amply satisfied in the neighbourhood of Naples. Every spot in the

Campi Flegrei became familiar to me. I repeatedly
ascended Vesuvius—once in attendance on the Princess,
who reached the edge of the Crater, and was fortunate
in witnessing a sudden explosion of flame with the
ejection of some large ignited stones—a pleasurable
excitement to one of her temperament, always courting
rather than shunning bold and hazardous chances,
whether of personal or political danger. These occasional
explosions from Vesuvius, with the more constant ones
of Stromboli, are the most active forms of eruption I
have seen, largely though I have travelled in volcanic
countries.

Accustomed to speak Italian during my journeys in
the Levant, and favoured in several other ways, I entered much into Neapolitan society. The families of
the Marchese di Berio, of the Duca di Sangro, the Duca
di Noia, and the different branches of the Caraffa family,
were amongst those with whom I lived most intimately.
Of the splendid library of the Marchese di Berio, and
that of another friend, the Archbishop of Tarento, I
made much use. I fear I might speak of myself as one
of the very few living who can remember the magnificent
Cat, forming the chief member in the household of this
venerable and kind-hearted prelate. The Cat and the
Archbishop, sitting together as they generally did, made
a picture in themselves—the former looking, according
to my recollections, the more austere theologian of the
two. I must confess to a very different associate in my
frequent visits to the Berio library. Laura di Berio,
the younger daughter of the Marquis, a rare specimen of

the peculiar beauty of Italy, and richly imbued with her father's literary tastes—proffered herself as my instructress in the reading of Italian poetry. Whether an apt scholar or not, my memory forces me to confess that I was a willing one.

I might well be tempted to dwell longer on these recollections of the four months passed at Naples as a time of singular enjoyment. It came to a sudden and compulsory end. The landing of Napoleon, now publicly known, and the instant preparation of King Joachim to march against the Austrians, made a change here as rapid and complete as the shifting of a scene at the theatre. It was in truth the dropping of the curtain upon a gorgeous drama. The days of revelry closed with a painful abruptness; intimacies just formed were broken, never to be renewed; and no one saw what lay in the future. At this crisis we departed very hastily for Rome, the Clorinde frigate being ordered to meet the Princess at Civita Vecchia. Since that time, now fifty-six years ago, I have never seen Naples again, though near to it more than once. I have been conscious of a certain reluctance to revisit a place involving so many memories of what has either changed or utterly passed away. If such feeling be a weakness, it is at least not an uncommon one, and hardly to be reprehended.

We found Rome in the same confusion and dismay in which we had left Naples. The Neapolitan troops were close at hand, and no preparation made to repel them. Flight was the order of the day, but under uncertainty how and whither. The short time we passed here was profitless in every way, save in the opportunity of revisiting the studio of Canova, and seeing under his guidance the works of art in the Borghese Palace. After a detention of some days at Civita Vecchia, we embarked in the Clorinde ; touched at Porto Ferraio—just vacated by the man who gave Elba a transient fame, and was then carrying fresh fire into Europe—and landed at Genoa, now occupied by some thousand English troops, commanded by my friend Lord William Bentinck. It was the third time I had met him in command of an English Mediterranean army. The family traits were favourably represented in the simple, upright, and manly character of this nobleman, translated afterwards to the government of our Indian Empire.

At Genoa, while war was sternly in preparation elsewhere, we passed six weeks of tranquillity ; scarcely ruffled by the rumours from without, and excited only by the arrival of fugitives from the Roman and other States. Chief of these was Pius VII., once more driven from Rome, and seeking refuge in a Protestant garrison. I saw him land, with several Cardinals in his suite, and traverse the City to the palace prepared for him, guarded by files of English soldiers. Almost every day subsequently we saw him pass the Durazzo Palace, where the Princess resided, in a carriage guarded by English dragoons !—a spectacle strange even in those days of strange events. Visits were reciprocated, as at Rome, between the Pope and the Princess, on both which occasions I was in attendance on the

latter. Soon after his arrival, I saw him in that extraordinary church, the Duomo di San Lorenzo, with a
numerous body of Cardinals ; where, after celebration of
High Mass, he visited the sarcophagus, alleged by
strange tradition to contain the ashes of St. John the
Baptist. The papal sanction given to such a history as
this, becomes a cogent disproof of the many kindred
beliefs to which the Romish Church assigns a traditional authority. Early in May we witnessed a more
splendid ceremony in the Chiesa dell' Annunziata—the
Pope, with fifteen Cardinals, assisting at High Mass—
the King of Sardinia and Prince de Carignan, the Queen
of Etruria and her son, the Princess of Wales and the
Duchess of Modena, seated in the same tribune—all
these personages more or less involved in the fatalities
of the time. After Mass the Pope proceeded to the
Negroti Palace, and from a balcony bestowed his bene-
diction on the kneeling multitude beneath—a spectacle
made more striking by its novelty to the earnest and
impassioned people among whom he came as a fugitive
This was the last time I saw Pius VII. in public. My
recollection of him was vividly renewed by Lawrence's
admirable portrait—perhaps the finest work of that
eminent painter.

I have much that is pleasant to remember of the
society at Genoa. I became intimate with many of
those who bear the names, and inhabit palaces, of
that ancient Genoese nobility, so famous in Mediterranean story—with several members of the Durazzo
family more especially. I found also a very agreeable

literary society here, and several men of science, who aided me in my different excursions along this magnificent coast. One of these excursions led me to the workings for coal at Cadibuona, a few miles north of Savona ; hitherto little known, but, as I soon saw from their geological position, not likely ever to enter into the general estimate of European coal.

From Genoa in the middle of May we proceeded to Milan. The Archduke John, representing the Emperor of Austria in his recovered rule of Lombardy, arrived there the same day. The ensuing week was occupied with various festivities—chariot races in the amphitheatre, masquerade balls, illuminations, and receptions. My acquaintance with the Archduke, begun at this time, was renewed two years afterwards at one of the Cheshire Salt-mines, into which we descended together—a poor spectacle, it must be owned, compared with the great Salt-mines of the Austrian Empire which I have since visited. His various scientific knowledge made the private society of the Archduke very agreeable ; but as Viceroy of Lombardy he was too liberal for the government he served, and was not long retained in this position.

During this second visit to Milan I interested myself in enquiries regarding the Pellagra of Lombardy. The observations I made as to this singular disease, in hospitals and elsewhere, were afterwards embodied in a paper printed in the ' Transactions of the Medico-Chirurgical Society.' At Bergen, in Norway, many years afterwards, I visited the Hospital of what has been called the Norwegian Lepra (Spedalsk), a disease very frequent in that country, and having close pathological relations to the Pellagra, though occurring under local conditions so widely different.

In going from Milan to Venice, we made short pauses at Verona and Padua. A rapid excursion from the latter city to the Euganean Hills showed me this curious insulated group of volcanic rocks and the tomb of Petrarch lying in a secluded village amidst them. That of Dante might better have been placed in a spot which once gave outbreak to subterranean fire. The Euganean Hills are much less visited than they deserve to be, though every traveller has them in sight in going from Verona to Venice. Even rushing past on the railroad, the eye practised in volcanic scenery can readily discern their character as such. They form in fact the northern extremity of that long line of volcanic action, stretching almost to the African coast, which cuts in twain the great basin of the Mediterranean Sea.

At Venice I remained a week only, having obtained Her Royal Highness's permission to return to England before the expiration of my year's engagement. Here again we found the ex-Royalists of Spain, fugitives from Rome, and carrying with them to each successive place of refuge the qualities, negative and positive, which concurred with the ambition of Napoleon in costing them their throne. I passed an evening with the King, Queen, and Godoy—an exact repetition of that already described at Rome ; marked, if possible, by still greater imbecility of the aged king.

I enjoyed however other society at Venice, and more intellectual in kind. At Milan I had made acquaintance with the poet Monti. Here I became acquainted with his contemporary rather than rival, Pindemonti; a man who blended a pleasing simplicity with his mild poetic genius. When Lord Byron finally left England, I gave him a letter of introduction to Pindemonti. Some months afterwards I received an answer from the latter, affording curious proof how much he had been perplexed by the *perfervidum ingenium* and wayward character of the English poet. No two men could be more diverse in their qualities. I presume that any intercourse between them must speedily have come to an end.

Leaving Venice, I returned to England across Germany by a route then new to me, since become very familiar, passing through Trieste, Vienna, Dresden, and Berlin to Hamburg. A short excursion into Hungary was my only deviation from the direct road. Traces of recent war were very frequent, especially in Northern Bohemia and Saxony, the scene of that extraordinary campaign, which ended with the battle of Leipsic. At a post-house near Prague, I heard the first vague rumour of the battle of Waterloo ; receiving it from P·ince Biren of Courland, whom I casually met there, and to whom the report had come in that mysterious way in which such rumours often travelled before steam and electricity became the messengers of man. It told merely of a great battle near Brussels—still going on, and the issue doubtful. I heard the history only partially even at Dresden ; and not in its completeness till I reached

Berlin, where I was present at the Church-thanksgivings for the victory.

This journey furnished some striking contrasts to the facility of modern travel. Driven to, and detained at the mouth of the Piave by an Adriatic storm, the passage by sea from Venice to Trieste occupied four days! In a light travelling carriage of my own, four days more were required for the journey from Trieste to Vienna. Three weary days and a night's travel, accidents included, were passed on the heavy sands between Berlin and Hamburg, and nine days on the passage from Hamburg to Hull. In the latter case, a certain compensation was afforded by being becalmed for two days on the Dogger Bank, amidst a crowd of London fishing smacks —a curious spectacle of maritime industry under the rudest conditions of bodily exposure—a still more curious spectacle of struggling animal life, dragged multitudinously in its many strange forms from the bottom of the sea. Such casual incidents, frequent formerly and often of much interest, are well-nigh lost in the mechanical and unbroken speed of modern travel, which shows little beyond the vulgar incidents of railroad stations, and the hurried transfer from crowded carriages to steam-boats equally crowded.

In connection with this narrative of my journey with the Princess of Wales, there comes another remembrance, six years later in date, which, though of more painful interest, I cannot wholly put aside, though I shall advert to it very briefly. The return of the Princess (now become Queen) to England in 1821, and the ensuing trial before the House of Lords, with all its antecedents and consequences, have become a page, and a melancholy one, in English history.   I was called as a witness by the Counsel for the Queen ; and was led by various reports, as well as by the manner of cross-examination of preceding witnesses attached to her suite, to suppose that much pressure would be put upon me by the Counsel on the opposite side.   The day before I was to appear at the bar of the House of Lords, I dined at Holland House, where the conversation, directed wholly to the events of the trial, was not cheering in the anticipations of the morrow.   The apprehension was needless.*   An erroneous report which, had it been true, might have embarrassed me, I was enabled at once to put aside by a simple and explicit denial.   Including the examination-in-chief by my friend, afterwards Chief Justice Tindal—the cross-examination by the Solicitor-General, afterwards Lord Lyndhurst—and that by the several peers who questioned me in sequel (Lord Erskine one of them), I was not detained more than an hour at the bar of the House, and encountered no difficulty which I was not prepared fairly to meet.   Two or three congratulatory notes from Peers present came to me immediately after the examination had closed.

---

* It may give some idea of the personal anxieties created by this trial, to mention that during its progress I was called upon to see as patients three Ladies, summoned as witnesses, and made ill by their apprehensions.   One of these only was examined, but this in a way to justify her fears.   I can affirm, notwithstanding one scene in the House of Lords, that the Queen herself was the person least excited or affected by the proceedings.

Nevertheless the whole procedure of this trial was painful to me, not solely as a national event, but yet more from my connection with the chief personages concerned in it. Though privileged to be present, I rarely entered the House of Lords during its progress. When I did, I generally had to note the difference between the reality of facts, and the aspect they derived from faulty evidence, or from the ignorance on various points of those great lawyers themselves who pleaded upon this evidence. Scarcely one of them had then acquired familiarity with foreign usages; and the want of this led more than once to curious mistakes in the conduct of the business.* Nor could I from my position be otherwise than cognisant of certain unwarrantable means of obtaining evidence, which, so obtained, was reluctantly used by the Counsel to whom it fell to employ it.

The trial was speedily followed by the Queen's death. Her whole temperament of mind, as I learnt from those in immediate attendance on her, underwent great change after the repulses she had encountered at the doors of the Abbey and Westminster Hall, on the day of the King's coronation—a painful spectacle, of which I was a witness. For the first time her spirit gave way. A casual visit I made to Brandenburgh House, where she

* Of the eminent Counsel of whom I venture thus to speak, one only (Dr. Lushington) yet survives, venerable not less from character than age. He amongst them was the favourite of the Queen. A remarkable fortune attended the whole number of these great lawyers. Six of them attained peerages; three filled the office of Lord Chancellor; two became Chief Justices; one, Master of the Rolls; two, Judges in other Courts.

L

then resided, was the first notice obtained of her illness, though acute inflammation of the bowels had already gone on for more than two days, without even attempt at relief. An imprudent exposure brought on the attack, and a further imprudence aggravated it. There was a strange sort of irrational bravery in the character of Queen Caroline, leading her to disregard all common precautions, not solely in reference to public opinion, but even where personal risk and suffering were concerned. She had certain talents and quick perceptions, as well as some really generous affections. Had these been nurtured by better education and by happier conditions of her married life, they might have left her a different name in the history of the time.

Seeing at once the urgent danger of the Queen's state, I sent instantly for other medical aid from town, scarcely quitting the house myself while she was yet alive. The symptoms had already gone too far to admit of more than partial alleviation, and never left a moment of doubt as to the issue. A prolonged life in this instance would have been an unhappy one to herself and unfortunate for the country.

I may mention here as one of the strange coincidences often occurring to a London physician, that I was called to Mrs. Fitzherbert as a patient at no long time after I had left the Princess of Wales in Italy. I continued to attend her for many successive years, seeing much of her also on other occasions. The contrast of character here was not less remarkable than that parity in one relation of life, which associated their names in the Court history of the day. I witnessed once, when meeting the Prince Regent and Mrs. Fitzherbert in the same room at Bridgewater House, that rejection of every intercourse on her part which gave origin to many anecdotes, true or false, on the subject.

On my arrival in England after this ten months' absence with the Queen, I found awaiting me a pressing invitation from Lord Amherst to accompany him to China, as physician to the Embassy about to depart for that country. This invitation, though offering some seductions, I did not hesitate to decline at once, having already mapped out my course in life and not wishing to delay or deviate from it. There was little in the actual history of this Embassy to make me afterwards regret my decision. It involved a failure as to the chief object in view, and a disastrous shipwreck on the voyage home.

One other tour, however, I made before beginning my London professional life—to France, Belgium and Holland. I saw Paris for the first time at a moment when it offered a strange and interesting spectacle. It was garrisoned by the English and Prussian armies—the former occupying the city north of the Seine, the Prussians the southern quarters; the bridges guarded with cannon. Entering the city, English soldiers were seen on guard at the barriers; they stood as sentinels at the theatres and public places, and were encamped in the Champs Élysées, Bois de Boulogne, and Montmartre. The day after my arrival I witnessed a magnificent military show in the review of more than 30,000 English and Hanoverian troops on the plains of St. Denys, where were repeated certain of the manœuvres of the battle of Salamanca—the Duke of Wellington commanding in person ; the Emperors of Russia and Austria, Blucher, Schwartzenberg, Platoff, and many other officers of fame present on the field. Lord Palmerston, then in the early stage of his political life, was among the English spectators of the scene. All this came in strange sequel to that long and sanguinary war which, under one ambitious man, had carried the French armies over the entire continent from Lisbon to Moscow, and well-nigh shut out England from the rest of the European world.

I witnessed another singular spectacle a few days afterwards—a line of Scotch fusiliers stationed along the galleries of the Louvre, while preparations were in progress for the removal of those great works of art which ranked among the most illustrious trophies of French conquest. In the course of the ensuing ten days, I saw some of the finest pictures, including the Transfiguration, taken down from their places in the gallery ; and the Apollo and Venus encased for removal under the superintendence of Canova. A sullen, and at times threatening crowd, not limited to the lower classes, filled the Place du Carrousel while all this was going on. The emotion swelled into actual tumult when the Austrian engineers came in to remove the Venetian Horses. The entrance to the Place was entirely closed for three days, and two Austrian battalions quartered within for further security, while English engineers aided the Austrians in their labour. Altogether the aspect of the French Capital

at this time was strange and exciting, blending together
the most discordant elements of the past and present.
Yet the whole seems to have passed out of the memory of
the Parisians with the generation that witnessed it—a
curious but common fact as regards events, even the most
momentous, which have not yet come within the domain
of history. In our own country will be found many who
are familiar with the political and other incidents of
Charles II.'s reign, while recollecting little of what intervened here between the battle of Waterloo and the
Reform Bill. Historical memory, like history itself,
abounds in incongruities, and this is one of them.

I renewed my acquaintance with Canova while he was
thus engaged in the Louvre. It was to him a labour of
love to provide for the safe restoration of these great
works of art, the glory of ancient Greece; and I watched
over his operations with interest and instruction. I met
him soon afterwards in London, at Lansdowne House
and elsewhere, but never again in Italy. Curiously
enough the successors to his fame at Rome have been
chiefly foreigners to the Italian soil. Thorwaldsen,
Gibson, and the three eminent sculptors who have done
honour to America by their works, are the names most
prominent in the recent history of Roman sculpture.
Thorwaldsen was personally unknown to me; but his Icelandic descent gave me an interest in him, much en-
hanced by those great productions of his genius, of
which the Danish Capital is justly proud. I never visit
Copenhagen without making the wonderful group of
statues in the Frue Kirche one of my first objects.

I was present, while in Paris, at a meeting of the Institute, and introduced to Vauquelin, Gay Lussac, Cuvier, and Biot; but I had no opportunity at that time of furthering my acquaintance with these remarkable men belonging to a generation of science now gone by. At this moment they were all paralysed by the critical events in progress around them, and the uncertainty of the future. How prolific of such crises have been the succeeding years of French history, even to the very time at which I am now writing! Scarcely two months ago I made the circuit of those ruined palaces and public buildings in and around Paris—the work not so much of the foreign enemy, as of that brutalized population of the capital itself, which gained sufficient ascendancy for a time to commit these and other worse outrages against humanity.

CHAPTER VI.

THUS far I have pursued my narrative with some regard to the order of time, and, for the reason before stated, with some detail as to those various travels which preceded my finally settling in London. Of the fifty-five years which have since elapsed, the retrospect must be a much more general one, both as regards my professional life and the other incidents blended with it. From mere medical anecdote, though it might enliven what I write, I shall, as I have before said, almost wholly abstain; while not scrupling to refer to those instances where my profession brought me into relation with men eminent in the history of the time. I have already spoken of this general design; but I note it again as a memento to myself, to shun as far as I can the errors into which autobiography is prone to fall.

In January 1816 I entered on my professional life in London, at the age of twenty-seven, with a fair augury of success speedily and completely fulfilled. My first residence was in Mount Street; but four years of prosperous practice enabled me to remove to the house in Brook Street where I have ever since lived; running deeply into a long lease by the length of my own life, while there is scarcely a house within sight of mine which

has not changed its tenancy four or five times over.
Time has endeared my own habitation to me, and I shall
never seek to change it.*

My early success was materially aided by visits for
four successive years to Spa, at the close of that which
is called the London season. This place (Spa) had
suddenly been revivified, as well by the memories of its
former repute as by the comparative facility of access
at a time when travelling was still a sort of tentative act,
strangely contrasted with the usages and appliances of
the present day. Nor had Spa yet been disturbed by
the rivalry of the innumerable foreign waters, especially
those of Germany, which now perplex the sick world by
their various medicinal or social claims, not always
blended in the most salutary way. Fashion and fancy,
quite as strong in regard to remedies as to other objects
of life, carry the periodical swarm of real or imaginary
invalids to many places less salubrious than the elder
and nearer springs of Spa. It is curious to note the
similar fashions of the Romans as to mineral waters,
implied in the sarcastic words of Pliny, ' *Medici qui
diverticulis aquarum fallunt ægrotos.*' It must be admitted that this phrase applies well to the usages of our
own time and country, as regards this part of medical
practice. But the fault is not on one side only. The
plea of health often put in at the end of the London
season, to obtain sanction for a watering place abroad

---

* My dining-room has a certain history of its own, in the tradition be-
queathed to me, that Burke very frequently dined in it when coming up to
London from his house at Beaconsfield.

instead of a country house at home, is one which taxes both the conscience and judgment of the physician.

The English as well as foreign society at Spa was large and singularly agreeable during each of the four autumnal seasons I passed there. That of 1818, coinciding in time with the Congress of Aix-la-Chapelle, was especially so. The proximity of the two places brought many diplomatists across the frontier, to the quieter amusements and better atmosphere of Spa ; among others the Duke of Wellington and Lord Londonderry, the Duc de Richelieu, Prince Hardenburgh, Prince Dolgoroucki, &c. The Emperor Alexander, the Prince and Princess of Orange, the Duke and Duchess of Cumberland, and two or three Prussian Princes, were among the numerous other visitors of this year. The Spadois were flattered and enriched by this concourse of Princes around the Pouhon Fountain, and by seeing three or four *gartered* English noblemen every evening at their assembly-rooms and roulette tables. The acting of Mdlle. Mars at the little theatre of Spa graced the season in another way—somewhat past her perfection, but still supreme in the parts she filled. She had that facile absorption into all her characters, which is so striking on the French comic stage. She was accused, and I believe with some truth, of being despotic and jealous behind the scenes. In this, as in other matters, the stage curtain is but a miniature of the curtain which separates the *seen* from the *unseen* in the great drama of human life.

I saw a good deal of the Duc de Richelieu in society ; quite enough to tell me that Talleyrand cared more for his bon-mot than for the truth of his sarcasm, when he eulogised the appointment of the Duke as Prime Minister—'Il est l'Homme de la France qui connoit mieux la Crimée.' The Duc de Richelieu was a fine specimen of what we are taught, rightly or wrongly, to picture as a French noble of the old school. He, the Duke of Wellington, and Lord Londonderry, walking arm in arm as I saw them at Spa, would have made an interesting subject for photography had the art then existed. But the Sun had not yet been enrolled as chief among the portrait-painters of the age.

I had a good deal of intercourse with Lord Londonderry at Spa, accompanying him in several excursions over the surrounding country. There was a certain nobility of presence and demeanour about him agreeable to the eye. Nor was this belied by his conversation,— always, in my recollection of it, acute and intelligent and in manner calmly courteous. This estimate, I am aware, is not that commonly received. The sarcasms of Moore's poetry, and one or two Parliamentary anecdotes, have clung to him with epigrammatic force. I may add that I never met a man for whom I should less have predicted the unhappy way in which his life was closed. Within a short period of time three of his contemporaries, all men of note in public life, came to their end in similar way.

I saw much too at Spa of Montrond, the friend of Talleyrand; if friendship be the word to denote the link between two men who lived in a common contempt of the feelings and fashions of the world, expressed with

a terseness of wit to which the French language gives
its most poignant form. The "*quoi! déjà ?*" commentary
of the latter, when Montrond was describing the *tourments
de l'enfer* which he suffered during some illness, was a
sort of exponent of the relations of the two men. I
never saw them together, but my later acquaintance
with Talleyrand told me of his mastery in the comparison. His wit moreover was the practical one of
having successively served three rival dynasties in the
highest positions of state, and taken at least a dozen
oaths of allegiance, while Montrond loitered through
life, leaving no mark behind and careless about it.

Many others of the politicians, exiles, semi-exiles and
adventurers thrown loose upon Europe by the events
of the preceding years, frequented Spa at this period.
One of the most eminent of those thus cast adrift was
Benjamin Constant, with whom I had before been
intimate in London. It was melancholy to see a man
of his ability passing the total day at the rouge-et-noir
table ; demaning himself by those follies of calculation
which bring ruin upon so many weaker minds. He was
manifestly ashamed of being thus seen, but the seduction was too strong for his will to overcome. There was
indeed in Constant a certain moral feebleness and fastidiousness which prevented his ever retaining long
together the position to which his intellects and acquirements entitled him. He reasoned and speculated about
events eloquently and ingeniously ; but had little faculty
either of action upon or resistance to them.

Professionally, as I have said, these four autumnal

visits to Spa were very useful to me, not merely as matter of present benefit, but as enlarging in the most agreeable way those connections upon which professional success in London greatly depends. Many private friendships too, formed here, remained unbroken in the further progress of life. But I am obliged to add that they have now, almost without a single exception, been dissolved by death—'*Hæc data pœna diu viventibus.*'

I gained a further good from these visits to Spa, by annexing to them each year some journey to parts of the Continent then unknown to me. On one occasion I joined Henry Drummond and Spencer Percival in travelling from Spa to Verona through the Tyrolese Alps, returning alone to England by Mont Cenis and Paris. Those—and there are yet many—who recollect the genial temperament and masculine though eccentric intellect of Henry Drummond, will appreciate the pleasure of a fortnight's travel with him through a country new to both. He had eyes and understanding peculiar to himself for all he saw, and language and manner as original as his thoughts. He was a man who could not tread along the highway of common opinion either in religion or politics, but his aberrant path was always pursued with honesty as well as vigour.

Another year in returning from Spa I made an interesting journey alone through the extinct volcanic country of the Eyfel, and the mining and manufacturing districts of the Prussian provinces on the Rhine, then recently restored to that monarchy and one of its most valuable possessions. In 1818, returning by Paris, I was one of

the guests at a dinner there which I have every reason
to remember. It was at the house of the Countess
Rumford, the widow of Lavoisier, a reminiscence in
itself. At the table were seated Laplace, Cuvier,
Berthollet, Gay Lussac, and Prony ; Madame Laplace,
Madame Berthollet, and Mrs. Marcet. Berzelius, whose
acquaintance I had made the same day at the Institute,
came in the evening. Such society, so assembled round
a Parisian dinner-table, was a singular treat to a young
London physician, and of its date and details I have
kept careful record. I had before slightly known Cuvier
and Gay Lussac, but to the others it was my first introduction. I sat next to Laplace at dinner ; and his fine
intellectual yet courtly face is still vividly before me, as
is the memory of a long conversation with him on the
geological theories and controversies of the day. He
brought to this terrestrial topic, insusceptible though it
be of similar proof, the same profound thought which
guided his researches in the Mecanique Celeste. With
Gay Lussac I had much talk after dinner on 'the doctrine of Definite Proportions, then recently become an
integral part of chemical science, of which it is now the
recognised foundation. Here my intimacy with Dalton
and Wollaston, and knowledge of the controversy still
kept up in Edinburgh on the subject, served me in some
stead. The topic indeed was one belonging especially
to Berthollet, who still clung in part to the older doctrines of Chemical Affinity. But with him my only
conversation turned on the actual political state of
France, on which he spoke earnestly but despondingly ;

—a condition of feeling common at that time to all thoughtful men, and well warranted by the various events that have since successively occurred in that country.

The eminent persons just named have now all passed away, but their labours form a large chapter in the history of science. It may well furnish food for reflection however, to note the mighty changes which the several sciences thus represented have since undergone —facts then deemed ultimate truths now merged in more general laws—theories upset and others framed— speculations converted into realities—lines of demarcation passed over—and methods of classification and nomenclature utterly changed. In these revolutions of the past we may fairly read something of the probable future—' *Quod hodie exemplis tuemur, mox inter exempla erit.*' Most things indeed, and scientific theories amongst them, must be counted as simply provisional in the present state of the world.

My narrative is so desultory throughout that I may mention here a much later visit to Paris, in the revolutionary year of 1848, which brought me into connection with another generation of scientific men—Arago, Leverrier, Dumas, Elie de Beaumont, &c. Of Arago and Leverrier I saw much at this time—the former especially deeply despondent as to the future, and speaking with great bitterness of the Provisional Government of which he had recently been himself a conspicuous member. Alluding to the bloody conflicts in the streets of Paris three months before, he told me that were such to recur, he was determined to put himself in the way of the earliest ball fired, to avoid further humiliation. His ardent and irritable temper shown in every part of life, and conspicuously even in his scientific career, might well have led to this end.

During this visit to Paris in 1848, I attended frequently the sittings of the National Assembly, agitated at that time by the speeches of Thiers, Lamartine, &c., upon the details of a constitution destined to speedy destruction. Scarcely a month before I had been in the rude hall of the Storthing at Christiania (now displaced by a more lordly but less picturesque structure), listening to the vehement speeches of Schweigard and Stäbel on Norwegian constitutional reforms, and the political relation of Norway to Sweden. It was one of the whimsical contrasts which have so often occurred to me in the tortuous course of my foreign travel. Nor is this my sole inroad into Scandinavian politics. In my last visit to Iceland, a few months ago, I was present at a debate in the Althing, the old Icelandic Parliament, on the administrative relations of Denmark to Iceland—a discussion which, as I have stated elsewhere, I could see to be temperately and ably conducted, though unable to comprehend its details.

At the close of the first four years in London, thus aided by these visits to Spa, I found my practice so rapidly augmenting as to justify me in defining more exactly my views for the future. It had been my original design to offer myself as one of the physicians of

St. George's Hospital on the first vacancy there, and with a fair probability of obtaining this appointment. No vacancy, however, occurred until I had reached a professional income which would have rendered such a position more burdensome than beneficial to me. And it so happened in the event, that at no time have I had official connection with any of the Hospitals or medical institutions which are usually the doors of ingress to London practice. If there were some disadvantages in this departure from the customary course, I felt them fully compensated by the time so gained for those other studies and pursuits pleasant to me in earlier years, but which I must have abandoned under the compulsion of an overcharged professional life, and which, once lost, could never have been resumed.

Thus authorised by early success, and wishing to pre-serve these former pursuits where not incompatible with professional obligations, I had first to consider how far my fondness for travel would come under prohibition. Looking back to the various good I had gained from this source, I thought it fair to anticipate the same for the future ; and I decided to take two months every year from my London life for this sole purpose, despite the cautions pressed upon me as to the impolicy of such innovation on the usage of London physicians. The mere phrase of '*going abroad*,' now become so familiar—perhaps too familiar—to our ears, had at that time much more serious import. There was a worldly risk run in my case, but I felt the object to be well worth the incurring it, whose health and pleasure were the assured result.

This resoution, carried into effect every successive year down to the present time, I have, as mentioned elsewhere, never found cause to regret. What indeed was innovation then has now passed into general custom ; and the physician who formerly snatched a hasty run to the Cumberland Lakes or Wales, as the sole relief to his yearly toils ; or merely exchanged London practice for that of some English watering place, is now found in the free and ample enjoyment of the Alps, Apennines, and Pyrenees. In some slight part my successful ex-ample may have aided in bringing about this change of custom ; but it of course mainly depends on the facili-ties given to every form of travel. In my own case the plan I laid down was easier of adoption, from a very large proportion of my practice being at the West End of London, and among classes of society usually absent from town in the autumn. But, with two or three ex-ceptions only, I have never exceeded the allotted two months of absence ; and never quitted London even for a day at any other time of the year, except when called to patients in the country.

These professional journeys in England were how-ever much more serious matters formerly, than they have now become under the appliances of modern travel. The electric telegraph and the railroad have in truth altered altogether the relations of the London physician to the rest of England. I recollect a journey in the severe December of 1833, when Lord Brougham, then Chancellor, begged, or rather compelled me to post down to Brougham Hall to see his brother James, dan-

M

gerously ill. This journey—unavailing for good to the patient, whom I found dying—cost me three nights of travel out of four. The only agreeable incident in it was a day passed with the venerable mother of the Chancellor, the niece of Robertson the historian. It happened to be her eightieth birthday. Her intellect was still sound and vigorous ; shown, amongst other proofs, by her clear apprehension of the peculiarities of that Son who has given fame to the family—a fame which, as regards himself, would have been augmented with posterity, had certain other qualities, deficient in him, been added to his eloquence and intellectual endowments.*

In another point I ventured from the beginning to outstep the ordinary rule of a physician's life, and with similar disregard of cautions suggested to me. My early travels abroad, as well as other accidental advantages already mentioned, gave me even in the outset of my London career a large access to society of very desirable kind. The question now pressed upon me, whether I should relinquish this, in some part at least, in deference to a supposed necessity ; or accept in full the advantage which circumstances had put in my power. The rapid increase of my practice speedily solved the question for me. I found that my habits as to society, maintained and extended, did in no way impede my progress, but

* On this occasion Mrs. Brougham told me that her judgment and advice had been adverse to her Son's acceptance of the Chancellorship. This circumstance has been incidentally confirmed by Lord Brougham himself in his autobiography.

simply directed it towards that branch of London practice most beneficial and agreeable to me. Had I not felt interest in my profession, the result might have been different, but feeling this interest, I never found cause to repent of the course I then adopted—one which has had salutary influence on all the succeeding years of life. For in pursuing my narrative, it will be seen how fortunately my lot has been cast as regards the society in which I have lived, both at my own house and elsewhere a good fortune continued to the very moment at which I am now writing, though under the condition of a totally new generation in place of that with which I was first connected. I can recollect at this moment but two persons now living—Lord Russell and Dr Babington—with whom I was intimate when thus entering on London life. Such memories and comments are inevitable as time goes on. Already they have often entered into my narrative, and I shall have frequent occasion to repeat them.

In the intercourse of society just denoted—and especially that I have been fortunate enough to maintain in my own house while never embarrassed by disparity of rank, it has sometimes been difficult and delicate to draw the line between professional connection and private friendship without impairing one or other of these relations this difficulty, one felt both by physician and patient, and the far weightier feeling of the disruption of friendships by death, may be fitly mentioned as the sole circumstances marring in any degree the happiness of my social connections. No attachments, as far as I can recollect, have ever been broken by other than the one inevitable cause, which for a time at least dissolves them all.

I have been speaking much of myself; but not, I hope, ostentatiously in my estimate of the advantages I have enjoyed. There yet occurred another matter, on which I ventured to disregard the admonitions tendered to me, even by persons of large experience in London practice. It was told me, and told very truly as a general fact, that there was danger to a young physician in gaining other repute than that belonging strictly to his profession—that the suspicion of literary tastes, or even of devotion to other parts of physical science, was taken as of evil augury for his medical ability.* More than one instance indeed had occurred to my own knowledge of failure owing presumably to this cause, where all other circumstances promised success. The question bore directly on my own case; since with my fondness for travel, I blended the inclination to certain other pursuits which I had taken up in early life, and was unwilling to relinquish.

Here again my early success served me in good stead. With a practice rapidly increasing, I could not feel it necessary to alter former habits, and abandon what was thus agreeable to me. And to my first resolution on this point I have ever since adhered. If indeed I had sought to reach that overwhelming practice which, being

* An instance came to my knowledge very long ago, where a man of the highest political rank, remonstrated with by his family for employing a particular physician, pleaded in reply that ' Dr. —— was so ignorant of everything else, that he could not be otherwise than profound in medicine.'

attained, destroys the comfort and often shortens the
life of the London physician, I should have found the
two objects utterly incompatible, and the former must
have been given up. But even thus early I had seen
and thought enough to dissuade me from such desire ;
and my feelings as to this matter were justified by the
absence of anything like pecuniary motive. From the
beginning my professional income had always gone
beyond my expenditure—usually doubled it. As early
as the fourth year of my practice in London it exceeded
1,200*l.* a year, and subsequently steadily increased.
The exemption from this most frequent cause of anxiety,
beneficial to me in many ways, was especially so by
enabling me to contract my labour whenever I found
that it became burdensome. This principle of restric-
tion indeed, after some experience, I put into a practical
form by resolving to keep my practice within 5,000*l.* a
year—a limit which, while closely approaching it, I have
never actually exceeded. To this resolution, aided by
my annual travel on land or sea in the autumn, I attribute mainly the health I have hitherto enjoyed. And
the general result has been that of a professional life
deviating in several respects from the ordinary course,
but to myself a prosperous one in every fitting sense
of the term.

The period of my largest practice was from 1830 to
1848 ; at a time of life well fitted for active work. The
experience, however, of two or three severe epidemics
during this period (those especially which bore the un-
scientific name of Influenza) showed me, in the heavy

and unwholesome labours of a few weeks, the penalty I should have paid in health and comfort by seeking to maintain this full occupation throughout the year. It is in truth as important to the welfare of the patient, as of the physician, that the mind of the latter should not be taxed and jaded by excess of work. The weariness of a long day, brought to the bedside of a patient, always impairs more or less what the highest professional skill and zeal can minister to his relief. The power of discrimination is lost or lessened, and practice too often passes into a hurried routine, unsatisfactory to the physician, profitless to the patient. This fact, fully confirmed to me by experience, requires neither explanation nor comment. It expresses simply what is the natural and necessary limit of mental power, and the wisdom as well as moral rectitude of acquiescing in it. The physician in full practice, like the lawyer in similar case, pleads the impossibility of contracting his work. There may be loss and difficulty in doing it, but with a strenuous intention and a wise regard to the future, it can always be done.

I have elsewhere spoken of my good fortune in going through a busy professional life with almost entire freedom from personal quarrel or controversy. I can recollect but one instance where my name was brought forward in a matter of public dispute—one of slight import to myself and speedily put to rest. So much of human life is embittered by passions or prejudices of a personal kind, that I have great reason to appreciate this exemption from them.

On the accession of the Queen to the throne in 1837, I was appointed one of Her Majesty's Physicians Extraordinary; and on her marriage I received the same appointment on the establishment of the Prince Consort. Of this admirable man, whose public and private virtues can never be too highly estimated, I saw enough in private intercourse to give me a full appreciation of those more genial qualities and accomplishments which, in the peculiar position he held, his upright mind felt it in some degree a duty to conceal. That fine passage of his writing, now published, in which he describes this position and his sense of the obligations attached to it, proves a perfection of moral discipline which very few can reach, still fewer sustain unimpaired through life. His high intellect showed itself, as I have often had occasion to see, in his quick and clear understanding of scientific as well as other subjects brought before him for the first time. The questions he asked in such cases were an index equally of his promptitude and power of thought. One of the fashions of this day is that of inter-parliamentary speeches. How few of these will bear comparison with the practical wisdom and true eloquence of those public addresses of the Prince Consort, which form in themselves a noble monument to his memory!

I indulge in this eulogium—to which, were it fitting, much more might be added—from a strong feeling of its truth. I was at Windsor Castle during the last three days of that illness which closed his life—a scene I can never forget.

At the close of 1852 I was honoured by the appointment of Physician in Ordinary to the Queen ; and a few months later (April 1853), by being created a Baronet. It much gratified me to receive the intimation of the Queen's pleasure as to the latter point through my friend Lord Aberdeen, then Prime Minister. Some years before (in 1841), the proposal of a Baronetcy had been made to me by Lord Melbourne, which I at that time declined, thinking my fortune scarcely sufficient, and not knowing how my eldest Son's career in life might be affected by it. Both these doubts were wholly removed when the question again occurred, and I could no longer hesitate to accept the honour offered to me.

CHAPTER VII.

THUS far I have been speaking of my professional life in its beginnings, and progress upwards. Passing at once over a long subsequent period, I may add still more briefly, that during the last ten or twelve years I have been receding from practice in a manner as satisfactory to me as was its commencement and earlier progress. The change has been a gradual one—depending very much on my own relinquishment of all that I felt to be onerous ; and this especially in the case of new patients, to whom I had not the responsibilities attaching to long connection and confidence. I have been spared thereby those abrupt changes and dissociations which often afflict the final stages of a successful professional career, and make leisure, when attained, a burden rather than relief.

Of later years, though charged with the larger provision for an eldest son which a Baronetcy rendered needful, I have had no pecuniary motive for continuing practice at all. My fortune had increased beyond my own requirements or those of my family. But the occupation, thus gradually modified as age advanced, became in some sort necessary to me. The habits of a life are never easily broken off—if suddenly, not always safely, as my medical experience sufficiently told me in the cases of others. I had myself enough of vital activity left to make demand for the employment of it ; and this employment was the more acceptable from its relation to the old professional connections of which I have just spoken, and which were still numerous and intimate. Some of these indeed went back more than forty years ; and among such I may especially mention the instances of Lord Lansdowne and Lord Aberdeen, to whom I was attached by constant friendship and correspondence during the whole of this long period.

This general outline of my professional life I might of course fill up with numerous details ; more interesting, it may well be, than the circumstances I have related affecting only myself. But I adhere to the rule I have adopted and already stated, of not indulging in medical anecdote further than through the notice of those more remarkable persons with whom I have been connected either professionally or by the common ties of social life ; and, for more obvious reasons, limiting this notice almost exclusively to those no longer living. Such curtailment of narrative necessarily involves a disproportionate reference to my own personal concerns, but I cannot conscientiously adopt any other plan.

The records of a generation just gone by must always however interest that which follows ; and the life of every London physician, of a certain standing, necessarily includes more or less knowledge of the eminent persons of his time, such in kind as may be described without any breach of professional faith. Their bodily ailments come

under his care—physically the same as those of other
men, and borne generally in like way—but now and then
portraying vividly in their progress those individualities
of character and intellect which have given to these men
their position in the world. I think it probable that the
peculiar circumstances, already related, under which I
entered into practice, have afforded me larger access
than usual, to persons thus marked for future memory.
I may count as among my patients at different periods
six men who have been Prime Ministers of England;
and much of other official practice has necessarily
accompanied this. Such practice cannot occur without
a certain knowledge of political events, and occasional
anticipation of changes not yet obvious to the public
eye. Several instances of this kind come to my memory,
connected chiefly with changes of Ministry at the time.
I refrain from mentioning details; nor would they now
in truth have any value, save in showing how largely
bodily temperament has its share with mental in the
government of the world; and how many anomalous
incidents of history may find possible or probable solution in the fluctuating health of the actors concerned in
them. When reading the histories of the great revolutions
of the world, as well as the biographies of eminent men,
such suggestions have often occurred to me.

The circumstance of private friendships being so much
blended with professional relations doubtless led to my
being often consulted on matters beyond the province of
the latter. In part also this was due to the character of
my practice—chiefly in a class of society where moral

causes mix most largely with material in affecting the health. In saying that I was thus led to give particular attention to such causes of malady, I do not mean to speak of this as any novelty in practice, since every intelligent physician holds the principle constantly before him, and acts upon it as a frequent necessity of medical treatment—substituting for drugs the more salutary advice as to methods and habits of life. If I have been especially sedulous as to this point, I trust I may add that it has not been without frequent good result to others, as well as myself. But it is a principle of practice often rendered inapplicable by patients themselves; many of whom are better pleased with a bald Latin prescription and the contents of phials and pill-boxes, than with the more simple methods of a well-regulated and wholesome life.

I have just slightly alluded to certain political incidents of my London life—chiefly personal indeed in their character, as I have never meddled with politics in any mere party sense, though from the accidents of early life, more connected with Whig families and society than with those of the opposite side. I may further speak here of a sort of semi-diplomacy in which I have been occasionally concerned in connection with my various journeys abroad, and especially those to the United States and the Levant. One of these occasions was that of the serious quarrel which ended in the Oregon Treaty. Having recently returned from Washington, where I heard much upon the question from members of the

American Government, I continued my intercourse by letter, under Lord Aberdeen's cognizance and suggestion ; and with the good effect at least of better defining some minor points on which there had been misunderstanding, and of aiding the conviction in America, that this upright English Statesman had for his sole object the just and peaceable settlement of the question. Again in 1859, when visiting President Buchanan at Washington, he put into my hands all the more recent documents regarding the San Juan question, including the instructions to General Scott for its provisional settlement. Here, as in so many other treaties, the omission of a few clear defining words provoked a dispute about this wretched little island, which mischievous people might have hurried on to the grave arbitrament of war.

There have been other occasions of later date, to which I will not do more than allude, where my intercourse with the British Minister at Washington, and the American Secretary of State, have in some slight degree subserved to negotiations in progress. I wish so to speak of these mere incidents as not to give them any fictitious importance. I dwell with far more interest on the belief that my numerous visits to the United States, and friendship with many of the most eminent men there, have done as much as is possible in the case of a single and private individual, to soften those feelings towards England which so many causes, real or imaginary, have occurred to disturb.*

* I may mention here, as an interesting recollection to myself, that on two different occasions, during my visit to the United States in 1863, I became the medium, without any direct intervention on my part, of recon-

Other accidents of travel have brought me somewhat curiously in the way of political events in progress at the time. Going to St. Petersburg in the autumn of 1830, by the quickest route then open, Lord Aberdeen gave me his despatches to Lord Heytesbury, conveying intelligence of the French Revolution of July—the first received in Russia ; unless, as asserted by some, the Emperor had private information a day or two earlier. Even ten days afterwards, when I returned from a journey to Tichvin, the event was either little known at St. Petersburg, or few ventured to utter openly their knowledge of it. The Russian newspapers, all officially controlled or inspired, brought out the facts in a fragmentary form disguising or obscuring the reality. I was at St. Petersburg again in the autumn of 1852, and saw much of our ambassador Sir Hamilton Seymour, at a time when the air was heavy with mysterious rumours of that impending war, which ended on the shores of the Black Sea. Passing some days at Moscow during the same journey, I found similar rumours everywhere afloat ; but whispered from ear to ear with that under-breath which despotism compels, and by which despots are often endangered. Nowhere is this lurid atmosphere of suspicion more oppressive than in these cities. I saw the Emperor Nicholas once only in this second visit to Russia. The change in the general expression of his countenance since I had last seen him, struck me

---

ciliation between persons of much political influence, who had in each case been separated by the heat of party conflicts, personally far more violent in America than they are in England.

as much greater than lapse of time could explain ; and this impression was confirmed to me by those who habitually saw much more of him. A certain harshness had come over features not naturally thus moulded, and with this, an impetuosity of manner which by mere chance I saw for a moment strikingly displayed.

Three years before this time, when visiting Sir Stratford Canning at Constantinople, I witnessed the prior aggression upon Turkey by Russia and Austria conjointly, in demanding the extradition of Kossuth and other Hungarian refugees. The excitement among the motley races peopling Constantinople, when the flags were taken down at the two Imperial Embassies, presented a curious scene. In no city are more diverse interests and feelings brought into action. Living as a guest in the hospitable house of our Ambassador at Therapia, I was cognisant of these events at each step of their progress. Despatches relating the demand made, and the conjoint sanction given to the Sultan's refusal by the English and French ambassadors, were committed to me by Sir Stratford Canning to convey to England ; and after a rapid journey by the route of Vienna, I deposited them in Downing Street even before reaching my own house. The prompt and successful issue of this diplomatic transaction strikingly attested the influence our Ambassador had attained, and so long ably and usefully maintained, in the councils of the Turkish Empire.

In the brief narrative of my earlier travels in Europe I have named several personages, more or less remarkable in their time, who came under my medical care. Without seeking to swell out a list of this kind, I may mention a few of those who in succeeding years of professional life in London have left strongest mark on my memory. Taking them as they occur to me at the moment, I shall be careless as to anything like order of time or connexion of the persons named.

One of the six Prime Ministers whom I have attended professionally was Mr. Canning, my relation to whom became that of friend as well as physician. It is pleasant to me to recall, through the haze of intervening years, my many conversations with this most accomplished man on literary or political topics—such conversations often occurring when he was confined to his couch by gout or other illness. One of them, turning upon his favourite poet Virgil, is more strongly impressed on my memory, from his presenting me at the moment with a copy of his own (a French edition in three volumes, 1754) lying on the table before him. He wrote his name, with mine, in each volume. This was immediately after a dangerous illness in which I attended him in 1825. There was a charm in his fine countenance enhancing that of his conversation, and felt by all who knew him. His voice well harmonised with these endowments—an influence itself always powerful, in private even more than in public life, surpassing that of mere beauty, and often surviving when all beauty is gone.*

---

* Various well-known passages show the feeling of our great poets as to this charm of voice. But it is strange how little this happy endowment is generally recognised in the amount of grace and pleasure it imparts to social

Other recollections blend themselves with the name of Mr. Canning—one of them illustrating a very curious form of mental aberration. In 1825 as I think, when he was Foreign Secretary and living at Gloucester Lodge, I was one morning called in haste to see a patient at Brompton. Scarcely had I entered the room of this gentleman (for such he was, and had filled a diplomatic office of some consideration) when he eagerly besought me to protect him against himself. He told me that a propensity to kill Mr. Canning had come upon him suddenly, and so strongly that he had taken these rooms at Brompton to be in the way of satisfying the impulse. But against this insane will (induced by some supposed official injustice), a sounder feeling was struggling within him, and for the moment gained mastery enough to lead him to seek for instant restraint. I of course lost no time in providing it ; warning Mr. Canning meanwhile to return to Gloucester Lodge by a different road. These strange cases of what may be called *duplicity* of the will are not rare in the long catalogue of mental infirmities. In lighter and less critical form such incongruities enter into the most familiar moods of character and acts of life : but even here they need to be self-recognised and resisted, to prevent their gaining mastery over the mind. The consistent and firm command over the will ranks amongst the highest attainments of man.

and domestic life ; and how little is done or attempted to educate an organ, which is susceptible of improvement even where nature has dealt harshly with it in the beginning. Quintilian counsels well on this subject, as on every other.

N

Another recollection again is strongly impressed upon
me. In February 1827, I was called down to Brighton
to see Mr. Canning, then suffering under very severe
illness—the effect, I cannot doubt, of midnight exposure
at the funeral of the Duke of York in the depth of
winter. On my return to London I hastened to Lord
Liverpool, to report to him on what he himself strongly
expressed to me as a matter vital to his Government.
Having satisfied his enquiries as to Mr. Canning, he
begged me to feel his own pulse—the first time I had
ever done so. Without giving details, I may say that I
found it such as to lead me to suggest an immediate
appeal to his medical advisers for careful watch over him.
The very next morning Lord Liverpool underwent the
paralytic stroke which closed his political life. His
pulse alone had given me cause for alarm ; but there
were one or two passages in our half-hour's conversation
so forcibly expressing the harassing anxieties of his
position, that I could hardly dissociate them from the
event which thus instantly followed.*

Six months after this time Mr. Canning himself was
no more! Succeeding to Lord Liverpool's place as

---

* I have a general distrust of all conversations or speeches reported after
long lapse of time, and have accustomed myself to try their reality by this
test of time, as well as by the length of the speech recorded. But the passage to which I here especially allude clings almost in words to my memory. Lord Liverpool said, ' Every morning I receive many letters on
matters of business. Some are indifferent ; some may be satisfactory;
some are certain to give me pain or anxiety.' The sort of emotion with
which he spoke this had reference chiefly to Mr. Canning's illness, but
might be explained also in part by what befell himself so immediately afterwards.

Premier when exhausted by recent illness ; and harassed by unceasing toil and turmoil, personal as well as political, from the moment of his taking the office, an attack of internal inflammation came on, under which he rapidly sank. I was called to him at Chiswick House where he was then staying; and found him already in urgent danger and under great suffering. I scarcely quitted him during the last two days of his life.* The difficulties he had in framing his Government became known to me through Lord Lansdowne, Mr. Huskisson, and Lord Dudley, of whom I saw much during this political crisis, in which they were closely and anxiously concerned. The aspect of the Catholic question at this' time, the temper of the King, and other personal causes, produced a partial disruption among the leaders of Opposition, and new official combinations which the death of Mr. Canning brought speedily to an end.

With Lord Dudley, as Mr. Ward, I had long been intimate both at home and abroad. The latter part of his life was clouded by circumstances which called upon me painfully in my double capacity of friend and physician. The organic disease of brain, eventually the cause of death, produced in its earlier progress many aberrations of intellect and temper, more striking from their conjunction with wit, learning, and intellectual power. Some of these aberrations, particularly those connected with his unconscious habit of *thinking aloud,*

---

* Mr. Canning said to me, as I was sitting by his bedside the day after I first saw him, ' I have struggled against this long, but it has conquered me at last.' (*Note Book.*)

became the anecdotes of the day. They first gave me
serious alarm when sitting alone with him in his drawing
room in Park Lane on that night during the progress of
the Reform Bill of 1832, when the mob committed their
outrages on his house, knowing him as one of the op-
ponents of the Bill. He showed no personal fear; but
the manner of his agitation betokened mental disorder
which rapidly augmented upon him after this time, ending as I have already stated. I think it worthy of
notice as a psychological fact, that his various eccen-
tricities abated much in degree during his tenure of the
Foreign Office; a relief he manifestly felt himself. The
exigencies of party threw him out of this Office, but he
quitted it reluctantly. He was a man singularly imper-
cipient of natural beauty or grandeur. I recollect to
have once been with him on the pinnacle of the Duomo
at Milan, without being able to extract a single phrase
of admiration for the wonderful view that lay around
and beneath us.

Though less intimate with Huskisson, I knew him
well enough to put due value on those high intellectual
and moral qualities, finely depictured in his countenance,
which were prematurely lost to the country. He was a
typical Englishman of the best kind. The first journey
I myself ever made on a railroad (in 1830) carried me
over the very spot in Lancashire where he had perished
but a few weeks before !

Another occasional patient of the same period, before
his election to the throne of Belgium, was King Leopold;
and the friendship with which he honoured me con-

tinued after this event. The first time I ever saw the
Prince was at Camelford House, where I passed an hour
with him beside the couch of the Princess Charlotte,
a few weeks only before the melancholy event which
closed her life. I saw much of him during the short
period when he stood marked as the future King of
Greece ; my knowledge of the country giving motive to
this intercourse. Happy for Belgium that the destination was revoked ! He was fond of reverting to this
subject. More than once, at Windsor or London, when
discussing the politics of Europe, he has asked me
what might have happened in the series of European
events, had this change not been made ? The answer
was an obvious one as regards each of the countries
directly concerned in the change—the collateral contingencies of the question were not so easily dealt with,
as may well be presumed from the changes which have
actually occurred in the political conditions of Europe
since that period. In October 1831, soon after his accession to the throne, I visited him at Brussels, and was
one of the guests at a great dinner at the palace. It was
the moment when the Protocols of the Five Powers had
concluded in sanctioning the march of a French army
for the siege of Antwerp. Among other guests at the
dinner were Marshal Gérard, commanding this army,
Count Mérode, Count D'Arschot, Marquis Chastelar,
and several of the more eminent Belgian deputies, M.
Rodenbach, Le Hon, Lebeau, &c. I purposely name
separately my excellent friend M. Van De Weyer, whom
I met here for the first time, and with whom it is my

happiness to say I have lived on terms of the closest intimacy ever since.

Another name occurs to me in connection with King Leopold, upon which I cannot forbear dwelling for a moment. This was Baron Stockmar—a man of rare probity and intelligence; qualities which he devoted, from motives of affection solely, to the service of the royal families of England and Belgium. I first knew him as one of the household of Prince Leopold; afterwards saw much of him at Buckingham Palace during his annual visit there; and once visited him with my eldest Son, at his modest residence at Coburg. His natural temperament and feeble health conspired to make him shrink from the world and from all public office; but his counsel was often sought for both here and abroad, and justly valued from its disinterestedness. The high regard ever felt for him by the Queen and Prince Consort was well warranted by his constant devotion to them and to their children. His life seemed to be chiefly concentrated in this object. His habits, dependent in part on his health, were very eccentric, and not such as might seem adapted to a Palace life. He had a singular aversion to writing letters; and even those addressed to him by royal personages, as I happen to know, often remained wholly unanswered.

Though I have known many of his family, it has never happened to me to see the first Napoleon; but I was consulted upon the disease which ended his life by his Italian physician Dr. Antommarchi, when he passed through England in 1819, on his way to St. Helena.

This was possibly done at the suggestion of some of the family in Italy. Though the materials for judgment were scanty and already dating far back, they sufficed to indicate the probable nature of the disease and its incurable character. The event very speedily confirmed these prognostics. Who can estimate what might have been the different condition of Europe, then and since, had the disease begun a dozen years earlier in that life which it finally closed! The history of nations may often turn on this single pivot of the health or sickness of some one human being.

My relation to his nephew—the remarkable man since Sovereign of France—has been of nearer kind. It began in the spring of 1831, when, without other intimation, I was one day summoned hastily to a house in Holles Street, and found there a young man suffering under severe gastric fever, and a lady hanging over his bed. This was Prince Louis Napoleon, with his mother Queen Hortense—just arrived from Paris, and the illness of the Prince seriously aggravated by the conditions of a secret and anxious journey through a country interdicted to him and his family. His recovery, the result of a good constitution and great calmness of temper, was more rapid than I at first expected; and they left England as soon as his ability to travel was well assured. I saw much at this time of Queen Hortense; and felt, as others had done, the charm of her voice and manner, made more touching in this instance by the illness of her Son, and the strong affection subsisting between them. She lived but a few years longer.

On the return of the Prince to London after her death—many events having occurred between—I saw him at intervals as a patient, either alone or with his French Physician Dr. Conneau, who has so honourably clung to him in all his changing fortunes. I dined at his house in Carlton Terrace some ten days before the attempt on Boulogne; without any suspicion of the event impending, though the party was chiefly composed of those who accompanied him in this ill-fated expedition—ill-fated but not ill-advised, as subsequent events have shown. Napoleon III. knew even then the value of the name he bears—a name which concurred with his own remarkable qualities in giving him the position he attained among the Sovereigns of Europe. My latest intercourse with him abroad was at Biaritz in 1862, when in the seeming plenitude of his power. But the seeds of decay were already sown in that Mexican enterprise, forming the first in a series of political fatalities. Forty years exactly from the time I first saw him in Holles Street I visited him at Chiselhurst—an exile again.

It has happened to me to have many Continental statesmen among my patients. I will mention only Talleyrand, Pozzo di Borgo, Guizot, Palmella, Bulow, and Drouyn de Lhuys. I might perhaps indeed add to these names that of the Princess Lieven, seeing the conspicuous part this lady once played in political as well as social life. I have known few women of such consummate tact and accomplishments, brought into such various practical activity. Her influence in the London world at one time was very singular. She wielded power both in Russian diplomacy, and as a Patroness of the Almack's balls, then the leading fashion or folly of the day. I am forced upon the latter word, by my recollection of the absurd tyranny which these balls and their patronesses exercised over the fashionable world at the time in question. Even as a physician I was often witness of the effects of this dominating passion, having seen more than one case defying medicine, cured by a ticket for Almack's opportunely obtained. I knew the Princess Lieven more intimately after her life had been embittered, first by the French revolution of 1848, and afterwards by the Crimean war—both of which events infringed deeply on the antecedents of her career. Like so many others who outlive a high position in the world, she felt strongly, and expressed to me frequently, the change thus attaching to her life. Her intimate friendship with M. Guizot is well known. Seeing much of them together at a critical period of European politics, it interested me to mark the contrast of the two minds addressing themselves in argument to the same topic— one generalising political life through philosophical maxims, a little too subtle perhaps for the uses of the world—the other bringing her eager thought and keen and well-practised sight to a much closer view of persons and passing events.

I first knew M. Guizot in 1840, when he came as Ambassador to England ; and I was one of twelve members of the Athenæum Club who gave him a dinner there, to mark our respect for his high literary eminence as

well as political reputation.*   Since the events of 1848
my relation to him has been that of more intimate
friendship and frequent correspondence almost to the
present time.   His works have all come to me from his
own hands ; the gift enhancing their value.   My attendance on his venerable mother in her last illness was
one link in this friendship.   She accompanied him in
his exile, and he repaid her by a devoted affection.

I have seen much less of his old political rival, M.
Thiers ; but my memory recalls to me one remarkable
evening I passed at his house in Paris.   It was in October
1848, and on the very day when the future Emperor,
then Prince Louis Napoleon, made his first speech in the
National Assembly.   The comments upon it by the
political leaders assembled at M. Thiers' party strangely
contrasted with the events of the following years ;
showing how little the real powers of the Prince were
understood at this stage of his extraordinary career.
M. Thiers evinced more sagacity when I happened to
meet him about three years afterwards, at the breakfast
table of the Belgian minister in Portland Place.   A
French newspaper came in, containing the report of a
speech by the Prince President on the opening a new
line of railway.   Thiers started up, declaring that some
speedy mischief was meant—wrote an excuse to Lord
Aberdeen, with whom he was to have dined, and set out

* Lord Lansdowne took the chair at this dinner ; at which were present
Lords Aberdeen, Stanhope, Northampton, Monteagle, Houghton and
Macaulay; Hallam, Milman, Senior, Palgrave, and myself. This little
record may have interest for the few survivors of the number, if they should
chance to see it.

for Paris the same afternoon. His prevision was verified. This speech was in fact the close precursor of the Coup d'État—itself the augury of more important change.

A French judgment alone can have weight on a question of eloquence ; but having once heard M. Thiers speak from the tribune (in 1848), I confess to having been less impressed by his public oratory than by the keen subtleties of his private conversation. It was however on a purely financial subject; and, though lasting an hour, interrupted only by the applause of the assembly. This power over the minds of men—the highest test of oratory—M. Thiers has maintained even down to the tumultuous time in which we are now living. It has done much to place him in the high position he now occupies in France.

I was very intimate with Pozzo di Borgo during the several years he passed in London as Russian Ambassador ; a place at his table being always open to me. His conversation, ever vigorous and poignant, epitomised amusingly the history of Europe for the preceding thirty years ; tinctured strongly throughout by that personal hatred for Napoleon, which dated, I believe, even from their school-boy days at Ajaccio. Nor was Pozzo di Borgo a man to forget or forgive the personal maltreatment he received somewhat later in a fight of factions there, when Napoleon was at the head of the opposite party. A favourite topic of narrative with him was the battle of Leipsic, the issue of which he always described as due to his efforts in bringing Bernadotte over at the last moment to the camp of the Allies—a statement confirmed from other and more independent sources. There is reason to believe also that his influence was much concerned in the restoration of Louis XVIII. after the battle of Waterloo. I saw Pozzo di Borgo later in life at Paris, when his mind was becoming clouded by those fitful imbecilities, which are always more painful when supervening on strong intellect actively employed.

My various travels abroad have brought me into professional connection with many other foreign Ambassadors resident in London. With the Duke of Palmella I was especially intimate during the many years of his stormy political life; and in the more tranquil years which closed it, I was twice his guest at Lisbon. On the death of his eldest son, the Duke sent to me, with a very touching letter, the 70 or 80 volumes of the Bibliotheca Classica Latina, which had belonged to this ingenuous and promising young man.

Of the Duc De Cazes I saw much while he was Ambassador in England. In his fine figure, courteous demeanour, and accomplished conversation, the qualities were obvious which rendered him personally so acceptable to Louis XVIII.

A much longer and closer friendship, beginning when he was in exile, attached me to Conte De Flahault, at a later period Ambassador himself; but far more intimately connected with England by other ties of education, marriage, residence, and the high esteem of all who knew him. Happy perhaps that his death preceded—though only just preceded—the last events which have cast so dark a cloud over his country.

I have been similarly connected with the successive Ministers of the United States in England, for a period of more than forty years. With Mr. Everett more particularly I preserved an unbroken friendship for twenty-five years ; visiting him six times at Boston, and maintaining a constant correspondence in the intervals between. My last visit to this virtuous and accomplished man was in 1863, after returning from the seat of war in Virginia. He was deeply affected by the incidents of this war ; in relation to which he maintained an honourable and consistent course throughout, often made painful by those disseverments of friendship which such events tend to produce. He died in the year following this last visit to him at Boston.

I was intimate and in frequent correspondence with another American of still higher eminence, Daniel Webster ; a man whom Sydney Smith aptly described as a 'steam-engine in trousers.' His massive forehead indeed strikingly betokened the massive intellect that lay within. He belonged to the earlier and higher class of American statesmen; though falling upon times when political partisanship and election trading had usurped so largely on the original institutions of the Republic, that he, as well as his contemporaries Clay and Colquhoun, were excluded from its highest office because they signally deserved it. I am half inclined to believe that the civil war might have been averted, had Webster's genius and masculine eloquence, as they at one time existed, placed him in a position where they could be of national avail.

It is pleasant to me to speak here of my friendship

with Baron Von Bunsen, whose genial and virtuous life endeared him to many more than those who could appreciate his great and multifarious learning. I had frequent intercourse with him on the particular subjects on which he thought and wrote so largely. He was an ardent lover of truth, but had a certain preference for seeking it through unwonted and obscure paths, not always opening into clear day, even to himself. A conception loomed before him of some attainable unity of religious belief in the world, and upon this conception he sedulously but unsuccessfully worked. The object may well be deemed a worthy one ; but not to be attained without many prior changes of human character and condition.

My plan of narrative restrains me from saying much of those still living ; but I would briefly notice my intimacy with M. Drouyn de Lhuys while Ambassador in England, from regard to his high intellectual character, and his extraordinary English scholarship. I have heard him at my own table rightly assign a couplet to Dryden of which others questioned the authorship. I have rarely known so passionate an admirer of Shakespeare, or one who so justly appreciated the profound philosophy of our great poet. He spoke of this to me as his best solace under any ailment or depression of mind, and I have known him repeatedly use it as such. I happened to be dining with him in Belgrave Square, and discussing a passage in one of the plays, when a telegraphic message from Paris interrupted us, recalling him immediately to France in reference to the Greek question then in agitation. He left London early the next morning, and it has never happened to me to see him since.

Having thus far departed from my rule of not speaking of persons yet living, I may say a few words here about another patient : whose political life indeed has come to an end, but whose name will still have a place in history. This is Jefferson Davis. I first knew him at Washington in 1856, when he was Secretary of War in the Cabinet of President Pierce : and a note made at the time shows me how much I was then impressed by his demeanour and conversation. He stood in singular contrast to the quiet and amiable man whom he nominally served, and really governed. It was three years later, when I was a guest of President Buchanan at the White House, that he consulted me upon his state of health. The following year, when again at Washington with the Prince of Wales, I became acquainted with Mrs. Davis—a lady whose energy is said to have supported that of her husband during the protracted and bloody struggle then so close at hand, though to the last moment unforeseen, save by a few who were mischievously concerned in the events which brought on the crisis.*

My intercourse with Talleyrand was chiefly at Holland House, where I frequently met him at dinner, a meal to which he came with his animal appetites keenly awake to enjoyment. His face and figure have been

---

* (1869.) In the spring of this year Jefferson Davis was in London, and it gratified me to be able to render some kindness to a man broken down in mind, body, and estate by the events of the preceding years. Political feeling can have no fit place in cases of this kind.

often described. If I were to speak of them as they were when I knew him, I should simply say they were indescribable. His portrait at Holland House is placed between those of Mackintosh and Romilly ; a contrast as strange as were the characters of the men. It could hardly have been mere casualty which gave it this position. His conversation also was cast in a mould of its own, very unlike anything else—short, pithy sentences, poignant in their sarcasms upon men and events, witty without effort or the assumption of being so. In studying Talleyrand—and it was a curious study—a comparison often suggested itself to me in Cardinal de Retz. Their intellectual and moral qualities were of the same general stamp, and attested much in the same way, though on a very different scale of action. Their epigrammatic maxims have the same peculiar flavour, and their ecclesiastical positions the same relation to the actual religion of the two men. The Cardinal, however, doubtless stands lowest in the comparison. The petty incidents and passions of the 'Guerre de la Fronde' were little fitted to dignify a public career.

The *bons-mots* of Talleyrand have been often recorded ; some of these indeed fathered upon him though coming from earlier sources. Wholly absorbed in the physical pleasure of eating, he spoke little during dinner, and little in the early stages of digestion. This devotion to the single real meal of the day he did not seek to disguise. Later in the evening his eloquence, if such it might be called, broke out ; and more than once I have listened to him until midnight with unabated interest.

His power of simple narrative was extraordinary. It was a succession of salient pictures, never tedious from being kept too long before the eye, and coloured by an epigrammatic brevity and felicity of language peculiar to himself. Two instances occur to me at this moment— one a description, sarcastic chiefly yet with some passing touches of pathos, of the deathbed of Louis XVIII., at which he was officially present—the other a vivid sketch of the several Marshals of the French army who gained fame and title in the wars of Napoleon—the latter contradicting in many points the current opinions, founded on the various histories and bulletins of the time. If I rightly remember, Marshal Mortier was the one whom he mentioned with greatest respect. I do not recollect ever to have heard him speak of Napoleon otherwise than incidentally, and with little commentary added. That he read his character truly and thoroughly cannot be doubted. That he had no love for him was equally certain. Political convenience only could have overcome the repulsion of two minds so incongruous in every particular ; and such convenience was, in fact, their actual relation in public life.*

If I were to seek for a strongly marked contrast to the character, figure, and speech of Talleyrand, I might

---

* I am told that the Memoirs of Talleyrand exist, and will be published at a period indicated by himself. But for this information I should have thought him a man little likely to become a journal writer ; and not caring enough for posterity to bequeath to it a history of the times in which he lived. If really published, these Memoirs will be both in substance and style among the most curious documents of modern history.

name Lord Sidmouth—a patient of mine at the same period, and whom I saw as such to the close of his long and placid life. His anecdotes of past events—and he delighted in giving them at length—were moulded in very different phraseology from those of Talleyrand. The personages entering most largely into these narratives were George III., Mr. Pitt, and Mr. Canning ; and very naturally so as regards the particular incidents which gave him the position of Prime Minister, and removed him from it. But I recollect nothing to alter the conclusions already formed as to that administration of Lord Sidmouth, which hung so much upon causes alien to himself, as indeed did most of the events of his political career. When he told me, as he often did, that no events of the day had ever ruffled his night's sleep, he described one particular effect of that temperament which protracted his life to nearly ninety, but left little else of lasting history to the world.

I visited him occasionally at Richmond Park, but more frequently at Lord Stowell's in Grafton Street —the latter visits the more agreeable, as including the society of Lord Stowell himself. I have a lively recollection of the evenings I passed with these two men ; widely differing in character and talent, but united by family ties, common politics, and a common love of port wine, which, excellent of its kind, was ever present on the table. Lord Sidmouth was the talker of the party ; but the whimsical roll of Lord Stowell's massive shoulder, when uttering some interlocutory phrase of dry humour, was worth more to the eye than any amount of speech to the ear. Lord Alvanley's description of him, as 'a conceited Muscovy duck,' had an amusing personal reality about it, felt even by those who knew his high merits as a Judge and master of international law. His house curiously illustrated the habits of the man, in its utter destitution of all the appliances of luxury or comfort. The furniture was never either changed or cleaned. Year after year I wrote prescriptions there with the same solitary pen—the single one, I believe, in his possession, and rarely used by himself after his retirement from public business. He had corresponded with Dr. Johnson early in life. Latterly he rarely wrote a letter. Of society, even legal, he had little or none, and he did not covet it.*

Lord Melbourne I knew long before I attended him professionally. This attendance—beginning when he was Premier, and continued to the time of his death— was interesting to me, in the observation of qualities of mind and heart rarely blended in such position of life. A clear and masculine understanding, lightened by great kindness of temper and genial humour, vested itself in language of almost rustic plainness. There was something of the *abnormis sapiens* about him in his power of reaching sound conclusions by unwonted paths —conclusions which often sounded like maxims, from

* A letter, written to Lord Stowell (then Sir William Scott) by Dr. Johnson, two or three months before his death, was given me by Lady Sidmouth. Not being a collector myself, I transferred it to the valuable collection of my friend Lord Houghton. I believe the anecdote to be mainly true that Lord Stowell visited most of the *shilling sights* of London, but did not go beyond this price.

the terse simplicity of their expression.   Singularly
handsome in the best English type, he was wholly
without personal vanity.   He attained and retained
the foremost place in political life, without ambition and
without party animosity.   Under the semblance of carelessness about men and things, and real carelessness as
to what concerned himself personally, he was deeply
conscientious in all that he deemed the interests of the
country.   Though he could joke about the making of
Bishops, and complain in somewhat homely phrase of
the trouble they gave him by dying, no subject, as I had
frequent opportunity of knowing, occasioned him more
earnest thought.   His devotion to the Queen, especially
in his later years, might almost be called a romantic
feeling.   After the paralytic stroke which first clouded
his life, this was even painfully testified by outward emotion, when any circumstance occurred to bring her name
before him.   His chief fault perhaps, as a Minister, was
that of too generously condoning what was faulty in
others.   I do not think I err or exceed the truth, in
speaking thus of Lord Melbourne, for I knew him long
and well.*

* A striking instance of the carelessness and candour blended in Lord
Melbourne's character occurred on the occasion of Faraday's pension.
The offer of this was unhappily couched in terms which offended the
feelings of Faraday, ever regardless of his own interests, but keenly alive
to the honour of the Sciences to which his life was devoted.   He refused
the pension, and stated strongly his reason for doing so.   Lord Melbourne,
dining at my house shortly afterwards, spoke to me privately of the error
he had unwittingly committed, and of his anxiety to retrieve it ; adding
that he would send me the next day a letter to Mr. Faraday, containing his
apology and explanation which, if approving it, he begged I would convey
myself.   The letter was an excellent one.   Its candour was fully appreciated by Faraday ; and the pension so justly due to this great philosopher
was finally, though not without hesitation, accepted.

The death of Lord Palmerston is still so recent an event, and his public character has been so amply eulogised, that I should not have touched upon his name, had I not been able to add one or two traits less generally known, characteristic of this remarkable man. One of these, of which I had frequent professional knowledge, was his wonderful power of *mastering*, I might call it *ignoring*, bodily pain. I have seen him, under a fit of gout which would have sent other men groaning to their couches, continue his work of writing or reading on public business almost without abatement, amidst the chaos of papers which covered the floor as well as the tables of his room. As a patient he was never fretful, but obedient in every way except as to this very point. And here indeed, though I at first remonstrated against these unusual labours during illness, I soon learnt that such remonstrance was not only fruitless but injudicious. To Lord Palmerston work was itself a remedy. The labour he loved 'physicked pain.' No anodyne I could have prescribed would have been equally effectual in allaying it—or, as I may better say, in lessening that *sense* of suffering, which is always augmented by the attention of the mind directed to it.*

Another point regarding Lord Palmerston, very little known, is the interest he took in all that concerned the Physical Sciences, and more especially Astronomy, Chemistry, and Mechanics. His knowledge on these sub-

---

* This curious point in Physiology is a subject on which I have explicitly treated in one of the chapters of my volume on *Mental Physiology*. See Chapter III.

jects, though of course general only, was very remarkable,
considering the many other and more pressing objects
which occupied his life.   He had not merely the desire
to know what of fresh discovery was in progress, but
also a singular facility in comprehending its objects and
results, even when altogether new to him.   I recollect at
the moment two striking instances of this quick apprehension—one, when I was describing to him Foucault's
beautiful apparatus for demonstrating to the eye,
and giving a record almost by minutes of the rotation
of the Earth—the other, when explaining to him the
method and results of the Spectrum Analysis, and its
wonderful application by Kirchoff and others to prove
the existence of certain well-known metals and other
elements in the environment of the Sun.   The questions
he asked on these occasions showed me how quickly he
comprehended and appreciated the facts I was relating
to him, though such as might well embarrass one new to
the subject.   Dining alone with him now and then in
the vacant season of the year, he always interrogated
me on these topics.   One or two other eminent instances
are known to me of this conjunction of scientific knowledge with political life.   But they are never likely to
become frequent.   The arenas are too far asunder to
allow of easy passage from one to the other.

I have elsewhere spoken of my relation to Lord
Aberdeen ; not professional only, but as honoured by his
friendship and correspondence for a long period of his
life.   No man ever brought greater integrity and sense
of public duty to the high offices in which his abilities

as a statesman successively placed him. If the energy
of a cheerful temperament was wanting to him, these
qualities made much compensation for its absence. I
happened to have some personal knowledge of his
conduct of business while Foreign Minister, and of
the singular, almost painful care he bestowed on every
despatch he wrote. The Prince Consort once spoke to
me of Lord Aberdeen in terms which showed how deeply
he respected him. There could have been no higher
testimony to his merits.

Looking back at some notes of December 1852, I see
that I passed the evening of the 16th with Lord Aberdeen, sitting with him till midnight. Early the next
morning he and Lord Lansdowne were summoned by
the Queen to Osborne to form a new Ministry, consequent upon Lord Derby's resignation. I was attending
Lord Lansdowne at the time under an attack of gout,
and he was unable to make the journey. I intimated
this immediately to Lord Aberdeen ; who, with the
honourable feeling which ever actuated him, delayed
going until he had communicated the impediment to
the Queen, and ascertained Her Majesty's wishes.
Ordered himself to form an Administration, I had occasion to know how importantly he was aided by Lord
Lansdowne in more than one difficulty which occurred
in constructing his Cabinet. The accession of Lord
Palmerston to it was not obtained until this intervention
had been actively exercised.

Without infringing on my rule of abstinence from
professional anecdote, I may briefly notice the singular

contrast of natural temperament between Lord Palmerston and Lord Aberdeen.   The inborn vivacity and optimism of the former pervaded his life both public and private ; rescuing him in great degree from many of those anxieties which press, more or less, upon every step of a minister's career.   He had a singular power of clear and prompt decision, as I had often occasion to know ; and was spared that painful recurrence to foregone doubt which torments feebler minds.   Lord Aberdeen habitually looked at objects and events through a more gloomy atmosphere.   He was wanting in that elasticity of body and spirit so influential in a public career.   I recollect, on one occasion, to have seen them as patients in immediate succession for several days together, when this contrast was presented under those strongly marked colours which illness more especially discloses.

The practice of the physician shows him indeed at every moment these strange diversities of human temperament, intellectual and moral ;—often concealed in part, and especially among the higher classes, by the outward usages and appliances of social life ; but disclosed, or even intensified, by the conditions under which he regards them.   Even where most obvious to common observation they scarcely receive due attention in the practical conduct of life.   The logic of one man's mind is not the logic of another ; and their feelings and tastes equally differ in kind and degree.   A rational allowance for these innate diversities of temperament might spare some of the conflicts and passions which disturb both public and private life.   But reason is not often or readily invoked in cases of this kind.

Though I saw but little of Lord Lyndhurst professionally, my intimacy with him, especially of late years, may warrant the mention of him among those public men of whom I am now speaking.   A *cross-examination* on such an occasion as the Queen's trial does not seem a probable foundation of friendship; yet this was my first relation to him, ripening soon into closer intimacy and frequent intercourse.   In the latter part of his long life (a family longevity) I usually passed an hour with him one day in each week.   I never knew a case in which the mental faculties, memory included, were so little altered or touched by age.   When approaching ninety, he exercised them keenly on the religious questions of the day, and especially those suggested by the volume of ' Essays and Reviews ' just published.   Some of these were obviously new to his thoughts ; and it interested me much to mark a mind, thus powerful and largely exercised on other subjects, grasping for the first time a question of evidence such as that of Scriptural inspiration, on which he often conversed with me.   Lord Lyndhurst's intellect would have been more fruitful had it been less subtle and sceptical.   He lost something of the real by his too keen perception of what is hollow or fantastic in human affairs.   He was more amused than disquieted by the foibles or errors of those around him ; and this even during his more active political life. The largest tribute I ever heard him pay to public opinion was the declaration that he never rose to speak in Parliament without some degree of nervous emotion.

Seeking among those men whom I have myself known, for parallel instances to that of Lord Lyndhurst, I might mention Mr. Thomas Grenville and the late Bishop of Exeter. With the latter I lived in much intimacy from his 50th to his 90th year. Meeting him frequently in company with Lòrd Lyndhurst, I had great interest in marking the points of parity and disparity between these two remarkable men ; each thoroughly understanding and enjoying the other. The Bishop of Exeter combined various qualities of mind, all remarkable in degree. His dominant faculties were better fitted for the judicial than the episcopal bench. Under the usually bland —perhaps too bland—and courteous demeanour of the Bishop, there lay a strong and subtle intellect, and a vein of astute irony cropping out on the surface whenever occasion presented itself. In mentioning these two instances of intellect long preserved entire, I should be unwilling to tax my memory for those others, unhappily more numerous, where great mental faculties, either from natural or casual causes, have fallen into premature decay.

I saw Lord Lyndhurst for the last time a day or two before I embarked for America in 1863. He was deeply interested in the events of the civil war there; and, though born in Massachusetts, a warm partisan of the South. He begged me to come to him immediately on my return, to tell what I had witnessed on the scene of warfare, as well as in the country at large.

Passing by his house a few hours after my return to London, I found a hatchment just placed on the wall. He had died ten days before!

The death of another old friend, Edward Ellice, occurred during this short absence of eight weeks. The preceding year I had passed a week with him at Glenquoich, that wild abode in the Western Highlands, where he annually collected a society which few country houses in England could rival. His own copious conversation was an epitome of all the events of the day. He too had strong personal interest in the American struggle. During my voyage home I wrote to him a long letter, relating my visit to the head-quarters of the Federal Army in Virginia. He was already dead when I wrote it!

It would be adding too much to this narrative were I to speak of the many others in the political life of the last generation with whom I have been intimate. I may briefly notice—and under the names they bore at the time—Lord Althorp, Poulett Thompson, Charles Grant, Labouchere, Sir James Graham, Spring-Rice, Cobden, Hobhouse, Sheil, Wilmot-Horton, &c. If I were to select from these names any for especial mention, they would be Lord Althorp and Cobden. The former I knew, not only in society and as a Minister, but also under circumstances of severe domestic affliction. He was an Englishman of the truest and best type, such as one might well desire to see multiplied for their country's good. His countenance pictured his integrity of mind. Silent in society, and without any talent for public speaking, he had the better eloquence of strong good sense, admirable temper, and high moral worth. Warmly attached to country pursuits, political life was a burden and sacrifice to him, which he threw off at the first possible opportunity.

I knew Cobden more especially during the last ten or twelve years of his life, and knew him also under circumstances of domestic unhappiness which weighed heavily on his mind without weakening it. Such ample tribute is still paid to his memory, that I need not dilate upon those remarkable qualities which have given him a place in the history of our times. I was present at a party at Lord Palmerston's on the sole occasion on which he appeared there, immediately after his refusal of a seat in the Cabinet. He had a certain feeling antagonistic to Lord Palmerston, which he never wholly surmounted. My own intercourse with Cobden was chiefly at my breakfast-table, to which he often came —always a genial and welcome guest. No meal better fitted for social enjoyment than this, if not impaired by those *hesterna vitia* of the dinner-table which so often sadden or unsettle the temper of the ensuing day.

Among patients or friends of earlier date I count four whose names come into connection with that of Dr. Johnson. One of these, Lord Stowell, I have already mentioned. Of the other three—Mrs. Piozzi (Mrs. Thrale), Sir W. Pepys, and Madame d'Arblay—I was best acquainted with the last. I attended her during the last twenty years of her long life; but her recollections furnished me with nothing new regarding the great friend of her youth. They were indeed at this time very vague, and she apparently felt little interest in reviving them. She lived in almost total seclusion from all but a few members of her own family ; changed her lodgings more frequently than her dresses, and occupied herself laboriously in composing those later works which retain so little of the charm of her earlier writings. Mr. Rogers was the only literary man who seemed to know of her existence. He liked to find out the literary recluses of a prior generation, and always dealt kindly with them.

These brief notices of some of the patients of fifty years' practice might be largely multiplied if made to include literary and scientific men of the time. Taking poets alone into account, I may speak of my relation both as physician and friend, to Walter Scott, Wordsworth, Campbell, Moore, Frere, Matthias, Sotheby, Praed, Luttrell, William Spencer, Joanna Baillie, Lady Dacre, &c. With Byron, Southey, Rogers, Crabbe, and Bowles, I was intimate, but not professionally. I saw Coleridge more rarely, and never took a place among the worshippers at his shrine. I recollect him only as an eloquent but intolerable talker ; impatient of the speech and opinions of others ; very inconsecutive, and putting forth with a plethora of words misty dogmas in theology and metaphysics, partly of German origin, which he never seemed to me to clear up to his own understanding or to that of others. What has come out posthumously of his philosophy has not removed this imputation upon it. I suspect his ' Table Talk,' as we have it in the very agreeable volume bearing this title, to have been sifted as well as abridged by the excellent judgment of the Editor.

Wordsworth, with whom I was much more intimate both at my own house and in his cottage at Rydal, also talked diffusely; but in a different vein of thought and phraseology. The latter part of his life was cheered by a redundance of that admiration which before had been confined to a few, and which he certainly did not undervalue. The phrase which Quintilian applies to Ovid, '*nimium amator ingenii sui*,' had its close application to Wordsworth. He frequently and fondly referred to his own poems, as if feeling that they had opened a new poetical era to the world. This to a certain extent was the truth. His fame had been clouded over for a time by the satire of the 'Edinburgh Review,' the supreme leader at that period of all critical judgments; but his poetry survived the satire and eclipsed it. This was not the only poetical judgment my friend Lord Jeffrey was called upon to revoke.

I happened to be in London when Lord Byron's fame was reaching its height, and saw much of him in society. It was one of those whimsical spectacles, periodically occurring, where an idol is suddenly set up by hands which afterwards help as assiduously to take it down. Though he was far from being a great or ambitious talker, his presence at this time made the fortune of any dinner or drawing-room party for which it could be obtained; and was always known by a crowd gathered round him, the female portion generally predominating.

I have seen many of these *epidemic* impulses of fashion in London society, but none more marked than this. There was a certain haughtiness or seeming indifference in his manner of receiving the homage tendered him, which did not however prevent him from resenting its withdrawal—an inconsistency not limited to the case of Lord Byron. Though brought into frequent intercourse by our common travels in the East, my intimacy with him went little beyond this. He was not a man with whom it was easy to cultivate friendship. He had that double or conflicting nature, well pictured by Dante, which rendered difficult any close or continued relations with him.* To his fame as one of the greatest of English poets I could add nothing by any tribute of mine. It is a fame which will be augmented rather than diminished by time.

My long recollections of Moore and Campbell are somewhat saddened by the gloom which came over the latter years of these two men, whom I saw in the days of their decline as I had done in those of their greater prosperity. The differences of character, national as well as personal, were strongly marked; but there were some circumstances in common, impairing alike the happiness of both—pecuniary need more or less constant, and a morbid sensitiveness to the opinion and admiration of the world. To this was added, in Campbell, a fastidiousness of taste, which gave exquisite point and polish to his poetry, but rendered composition laborious to him, even in those shorter pieces which seem

---

* Contra miglior voler, voler mal pugna.

struck off in the fervour of the moment, and by which he will be best remembered hereafter. Moore had more wit, ease, and elasticity, and with his Irish temperament better confronted the cares of life. But he too endured the heavy penalty, common to so many, of fame and fashion gradually passing away—a change which few can bear with equanimity. His Journals curiously indicate what I repeatedly witnessed in my own house and elsewhere, his morbid sensitiveness, when singing his Irish Ballads, to the effect they produced on those around him. In the most touching passages his eye was wandering round the room, scrutinising jealously the influence of his song.

Among the poets just named, Rogers was in many respects the most conspicuous in London society, and this for a period of more than half a century. Wealthy, unmarried, highly cultivated in all matters of literature and art, his conversation seasoned with anecdote and personal sarcasms uttered in a curious sepulchral voice, he gained and kept a higher place than his poetry alone would have procured for him. He was the arbiter in many of the literary controversies and quarrels of his day. His dinner-table—the *blanda conciliatrix* in so many social discords—ministered well to this object. In society his most severe sarcasms were often hidden under honeyed phrases ; leaving them obvious to others, while undetected by those whose foibles he assailed. There was foundation for the remark that a note from Rogers generally conveyed some indirect satire on the person to whom it was addressed—the more flattery on the surface, the more gall underneath. He could be and was ever generous to poverty and real distress, but intolerant to all that presented itself in social rivalry to himself. The usurpation by others of talk at a dinner table, or an interruption to one of his own anecdotes, was sure to provoke some access of bitterness bitterly expressed. These feelings increased with increasing age. They were somewhat curiously modified in the distrust with which he latterly regarded his own memory—rarely venturing upon an anecdote without a *caveat* as to his having told it before. He long survived most of his contemporaries of middle life, and all those who, in retaliation for his sarcasms, were wont to spend their wit on his death-like physiognomy. I never could learn why so little has been given to the world of those Journals of which he used often to read portions to his friends, and which bore on the face of them the characteristic marks of keen observation and minute fidelity.

His dinners were fashioned in the same artistic mould as his poetry—the society small and select, the cookery superlative ; no candles on the table, but light thrown from shaded lamps on the pictures around the room, each a small but consummate gem of art. As a specimen of these dinner parties, I can remember one where I met Walter Scott, Southey, Wordsworth, Crabbe, Luttrell, Lockhart, and I think my friend Henry Taylor, now the sole survivor of the number.

While speaking of literary dinners, my memory carries me back to those of Mr. Thomas Hope, curiously contrasted with Mr. Rogers's dinners in the character of

P

the host, but amongst the most agreable I have known in London life. The philosophic thought and various learning which Mr. Hope possessed were conjoined with a gentle simplicity of manner, giving him a great charm in society. My own recent travels in the East enabled me to appreciate the truthful accuracy of description in his 'Anastasius,' as well as the power of narrative and delineation of character which made this book so popular at the time.

I will not seek excuse in the garrulousness of age for these and other similar details of former life, but would more willingly regard them as fitting remembrances of men who belonged in one way or other to the history of their time, and upon some of whom posterity may still have to pronounce its judgment. If this judgment is now and then faulty in its oblivion of true genius, it redeems the error by suppressing what are false titles to future fame.

CHAPTER VIII.

I GO on now to other incidents of my own life, mixing them, as I have already done, with notices of the persons with whom I have lived in relations of friendship or intimacy. Without care as to the order of time, I shall narrate these incidents very much as they occur to my recollection, and first indeed reverting to some of very early date.

In 1816 I became a Fellow of the Royal Society; my election thus early in life being due to my travels in Iceland and Greece, and to my acquaintance with Sir Joseph Banks (then a supreme power in the Society), as well as with Sir H. Davy, whose recent discoveries had raised him into high eminence. I was received as a Fellow on the same evening as Lord Byron—his sole appearance at the Royal Society, to which he had few affinities of knowledge or taste. I have three times held the office of Vice-President; and I am now, since the death of my admirable friend Sir John Herschel, the eldest in date of the existing Fellows of the Royal Society. It is a striking proof of the elastic expansion of physical science in all its various branches, that notwithstanding the detachment of so many scientific societies from this parent stem, its 'Transactions' still record

discoveries as numerous and important as at any period
of its history. This indeed must still continue ; since
every discovery made discloses new objects of research,
and new methods of attaining them. The methods
themselves may often be ranked among the greatest discoveries and most signal monuments of human genius.

I was a frequent attendant at the meetings of the
Fellows of the Society on Sunday Evenings, at the
house of Sir Joseph Banks, in Soho Square. It was a
remarkable assemblage of men of a generation now gone
by—but a generation which may claim parentage to the
researches out of which their successors have evolved
such wonderful results. Among those most constantly
present were Cavendish, Wollaston, Davy, Young,
Chenevix, Davies Gilbert, Pond, Prout, Robert Brown,
Tenant, Hatchett, Warburton, &c. Sir W. Herschel I
have seen there, but more rarely. Dalton also, whom I
had well known before in his rude laboratory of broken
bottles and other uncouth apparatus at Manchester,
appeared occasionally—an individuality in himself, apart
from the Quaker garb he wore. His relations to the
Atomic theory will ever leave him a marked place in the
history of physical science.

Two striking figures at these meetings were Cavendish
and Wollaston—the former the shyest and most taciturn
of men ; listening intently when discussion was going
on, but never taking part in it ; and shrinking out of
sight if reference were made to himself or his own researches—Wollaston, sternly logical and sceptical, listening to others as if ever ready to refute or rebuke, and

generally doing so by pungent questions to which few could venture to reply. I have often known a plausible theory, uttered by some one unconscious of Wollaston's presence, suddenly upset by two or three of these abrupt questions or comments. To the mere pretence of science he showed no mercy. The habitual scepticism of his mind was, however, a hindrance to his own scientific career. This was strikingly shown in the circumstances attending his discovery of the metal Palladium ; and at a later time in his relation to the greater discovery of the Electro-Magnetic rotation. Though the first to denote the dark lines in the Solar Spectrum, the germ of so many later researches, he did not himself carry the observation further. That aid which hypothesis, duly limited, renders to experimental enquiry, he unduly disdained and put aside. He would have accomplished more had he doubted less.

At these parties in Soho Square, the youthful and more elastic genius of Davy came in striking contrast to the inflexibility of Wollaston and the *umbratilis vita* and hereditary taciturnity of Cavendish. His early successes in science had emboldened a mind naturally ardent and speculative ; and I well remember the eagerness with which men clustered around him to listen to his eloquent anticipations of future progress, many of these now more than fulfilled. His Lectures at the Royal Institution, novel and earnest in manner, and invigorated by the succession of discoveries they recorded, brought crowds of admiring hearers. Admiration, indeed, derived from other sources than those of science was one of several concurrent influences on Davy's natural character, altering it disadvantageously in several respects.   I knew him intimately throughout the greater part of his career ; and with melancholy interest through those stages of decline sequent on his first paralytic attack.   I saw him under this seizure a few hours after its occurrence, and when he was hardly yet aware of its nature or import.   The peculiarities of his mind, his genius and irritability, were strikingly marked when the consciousness of the event came fully upon him.

So in a different way were those of Wollaston, under another form of cerebral disease, which, though less sudden in its beginning, ended more speedily in death. Watching over his latter days with Sir B. Brodie, it was matter of deep interest to us to observe his philosophical mind taking calm but careful note of its own decay— the higher faculties, which were little if at all impaired, occupied in testing by daily experiments of his own suggestion, the changes gradually taking place in the functions of the senses, the memory, and the voluntary power.   Diagrams and figures drawn on a board before him were among the methods he thus employed.   He had manifestly much interest, if not indeed a certain pleasure, in detecting the changes going on and in describing them to us.   He would admit no interpretation of them save in reference to that final change which he constantly and calmly kept in view.   It was a self-analysis of mind carried on to the last moments of life.

Dr. Young, again, stood in singular contrast to each of the remarkable men just mentioned.   His profound and very various knowledge was concealed under a certain spruceness of dress, demeanour, and voice, which strangely contradicted his Quaker origin, and perplexed those who had known him only from his scientific fame. I have seen the discoverer of some of the grandest and most occult laws of Light loitering with ladies in a fashionable shop of Bond Street, helping them in the choice of ribbons and other millinery. But what might hastily be deemed affectation was in Dr. Young not really such, but genuine courtesy and kindness of heart. My attachment to him gave me much interest in the valuable Memoir of his life by the late Dean of Ely, than whom no man was better able to appreciate his scientific achievements. These had been obscured for many years by an article of Lord Brougham's on his discoveries in the 'Edinburgh Review'—an article to which the term *erroneous* is the mildest that can be applied. They were eventually restored to their proper place in the annals of Science, by French philosophers succeeding in the same line of research. While interwoven with every part of the Theory of Light, they collaterally illustrate many others of the great physical problems of the Universe.*

Sir Joseph Banks himself was necessarily a very conspicuous personage in these parties at his house. Seated

---

* Sir J. Herschel speaks of 'the sagacity which would have done honour to Newton,' shown by Dr. Young in his discovery of the mode of propagation of luminous waves by transverse vibrations through the ether of space. It was at the Royal Institution that he first announced that essential physical connection between colours, and the organ of sense receiving them, which is now recognised as a fundamental principle in all these enquiries. I have often wondered that the *Eriometer* of Dr. Young has not been brought into some use at a time when atoms and molecules enter so largely into physical research.

and wheeled about in his arm-chair—his limbs helplessly knotted with gouty tumours—speaking no other language than English—and carrying his scientific knowledge little beyond the domain of Natural History, he nevertheless looked the governing power of the Royal Society, and was such in reality. I had frequent occasion to notice the strong impression his aspect and demeanour made upon foreigners—men of science and others—who came over to England at this period of renewed Continental intercourse. It is less paradoxical than it may seem, to say that this impression was strengthened by the very fact of his not speaking any foreign language. Silence often carries more weight with it than speech, and especially where the latter is encumbered by the effort to find words for its object. The intellect here becomes the slave of its instrument, and thought and argument are lost in the struggle to give them right expression. Sir Joseph Banks, silent in his chair, was more imposing than he would have been if exchanging imperfect phrases, whether of science or courtesy, with the strangers who came to visit him.

If this house gave scientific repute to the now deserted region of Soho Square, that of Payne Knight, close at hand, gave it repute for classical learning, art, and luxury. The dinners at this house were curious illustrations of its owner—the consummate scholar, the sensualist, and the sceptic.* I never dined with him without finding a large

---

* The Prolegomena to Payne Knight's Homer may rank as one of the most beautiful pieces of modern Latinity, and excellent, moreover, in its discussion of various points in the Homeric controversies.

dish of lampreys; and half a dozen learned men feeding on this and the other various luxuries of his table, with a relish which learning generally seems in no sort to impair. I knew Payne Knight before I went to Greece, and was well acquainted with his Cabinet of Bronzes, then the finest private collection in England. Among the most beautiful of these were the two Jupiters and an Apollo, reported to have been originally procured from Paramithia, a town of Epirus almost unknown to travellers. Mr. Knight urged me, if I came near this place, to make diligent enquiry on his behalf as to other possible treasures of like kind. In prosecuting a long and fruitless search after the site of the Oracle of Dodona, I twice passed through Paramithia, and pressed the enquiry in every way open to me, but wholly without success. Some residence on the spot is usually needed in such researches; and for this, a solitary traveller in a wild country, I had no time or means then at my disposal.

My acquaintance with Davy early in life gave me also an early connection with the Royal Institution, and with that laboratory which gained its first fame from his discoveries—a fame largely augmented by the genius and labours of Faraday, and well sustained by the eminent men who, as Professors of the Institution, now work on the same spot. More than sixty years have elapsed since I saw in the theatre there the minute globules of the alkaline metals, then first evolved in their elementary form; and witnessed the beautiful experiments by which Davy illustrated those relations between chemical actions and electricity, the foundation of so many ulterior discoveries. At a later time, in the same place, Faraday showed to me and other friends the small luminous spark which he had just succeeded in eliciting from the Magnet—the feeble precursor of those marvellous torrents of electricity which are now procured from the same source by methods as wonderful as the phenomena they produce. But a short time ago I saw once again on the shelves of the Institution the simple apparatus, devised by himself, through which he obtained this first result, the germ of so many others. Looking at what these results have been, there is grandeur in the very simplicity of their origin.*

The interest I have long felt in the labours and fame of the Royal Institution has become of late years more direct and personal, from the honour of its Presidency having been conferred upon me on the death of the Duke of Northumberland. Thinking it a point of chief importance to maintain the high character of the Insti-

---

* I write this a short time only after the death of Faraday. His name, even after his active labours had ceased, ennobled the Royal Institution both at home and abroad—a name scarcely more eminent from the great discoveries attached to it than from those private virtues and affections which endeared him to all who knew him. His love for science was as pure as all his other affections, wholly unalloyed by jealousy, seeking only for truth. His earnestness and natural eloquence as a lecturer will ever be remembered by those, young as well as old, who crowded to listen to him in that building which was his home for more than fifty years. The infirmity which came upon him during the last year or two of his life, touched not the moral part of his nature, which remained unaltered to the very last. To the tributes paid to Faraday's memory by some of the most eminent continental philosophers, must be added the excellent record of his life in the volume of Dr. Bence Jones.

tution as a school of scientific research, I have sought, in conjunction with others (and very especially with the aid of my friend Dr. Bence Jones), to establish a Research Fund, applicable mainly to the objects of the Laboratory. This aim has been well fulfilled ; and I hold a confident belief that our Laboratory and the eminent men who now work in it, will continue, as heretofore, to furnish discoveries for the Lecture Theatre above, and for more lasting record in the 'Transactions of the Royal Society,' which have already drawn so largely from this source. Every great discovery is the parent of many others; and the objects and aims of science are both enlarged and better defined by each successive attainment.

All periods have their particular fashions and foibles as well as higher characteristics. One belonging to the present time is that of accumulating literary and scientific titles, and crowding them after names not always well qualified to bear these appendages. The capital letters of the alphabet are called upon to do onerous duty in recording such titles. An excessive multiplication of Societies of every denomination and object, has indeed furnished facile food to this vanity—hurtful only in depriving such distinctions of their just and appropriate value. Honours, unfitly or too profusely bestowed, inflict injustice on those higher and rarer endowments which are the property of posterity as well as of their own age. I have partaken with others of these titles, foreign as well as English, coming to me at different times—the foreign made somewhat numerous by my various travels abroad. In 1847 I received the degree of LL.D from Cambridge in Massachusetts, of which University my friend Mr. Everett was at that time the President. In 1856, at the Oxford Commemoration, I received the degree of D.C.L. concurrently with several distinguished associates in the honour conferred—the Crown Prince of Prussia, the Prince of Baden, Lord Clarendon, Lord Elgin, and Lord Lyons. The Prince Consort was present on the occasion with his Son-in-law, a Prince whose admirable qualities have been signally marked in the extraordinary events of the last few years. . . . It was very agreeable to me to be elected, a few years later, one of the five Honorary Members of the Royal Academy : my present colleagues in this honourable position being Lord Stanhope, the Bishop of Winchester, and the Dean of Westminster. The deaths of Lord Macaulay and Mr. Hallam had left vacancies in the number, which the Dean of St. Paul's and I were elected to fill up. Another vacancy has just been created by the death of Mr. Grote.

The death of Dean Milman followed but too soon after his election ; an event deeply regretted by every one who knew him—by few more than by myself. The qualities of Dean Milman's mind, intellectual and moral, were such as to engage the affections of his friends even more than their admiration. Without noting his other and various works, the ' History of Latin Christianity ' would alone give him high and merited rank in English literature. As a writer he ever clung with masculine fidelity to what he believed to be truth. His eldest Son was with me at Trieste, on our way to

Dalmatia, when recalled by telegram announcing the paralytic stroke which soon afterwards closed his father's life. I myself went on alone to the magnificent coasts and isles of the ancient Illyria, but returned to England just in time to see my excellent friend once again.*

It is pleasant to me, though here also mingled with sorrow for many lost friends, to refer to another Institution, as it may rightly be called, with which I have been associated for the last thirty years. This is 'The Club' —emphatically so named—the creation, more than a century ago, of Johnson, Burke, Sir Joshua Reynolds, Goldsmith, Garrick, &c., and maintained ever since with undiminished reputation. At the Centenary dinner in 1864 (at which twenty-six members were present out of the total number of thirty-five) our treasurer at that

---

* Speaking in a former page of the *void places* in European travel, I might with some reason have included Dalmatia in the number, Spalato, Ragusa, and the Gulf of Cattaro might, indeed, alone suffice to invite the traveller to this grand mountain coast—the seat still of a hardy and intrepid race, well representing those ancient Illyrians who so long resisted the encroachments of Roman power. The Gulf of Cattaro was the chief scene of an insurrection against the Austrian rule, breaking out just after my visit to this wonderful spot three years ago. By an odd coincidence, my journey of the next year brought me in certain proximity to the Red River, but a few weeks before the insurrection which threatened the existence of this remote member of our Colonial Empire. Happening to mention this to Mr. Gladstone, he commented upon it by the very appropriate question, ' Pray, Sir Henry, may I ask what is your direction of travel this year?' I had not then fixed it; but it did turn out to be Jamaica; a colony still haunted by a certain fear—utterly groundless as I believe—of negro insurrection. The Dissolution of the House of Assembly, the wisdom of the Governor, and the reviving prosperity of the Island, are happily guarantees against any such event.

time, Dean Milman, produced a printed list of the
members of the Club from its foundation to the present
time, numbering 150 exactly—a document gathered from
those very curious volumes, which give written record
also of the persons present at each successive dinner
during this long period.* As a series of autographs
thus grouped together, these volumes are probably
unique. A formula which Mr. Gibbon suggested for
announcing the fact of his election to a new member is
still scrupulously maintained. It speaks of the *honour*
done to him in being admitted to the Club. Since the
time when I received this honour, in 1840, very many
indeed we have had to lament, removed by death—men
who gave to the Club the reflection of their own eminence, and were themselves warmly attached to it. I
may mention among the number, Lord Lansdowne,
Macaulay, Hallam, Lord Aberdeen, Lord Holland,
Lord Clarendon, Bishop Blomfield, Bishop Coplestone,
Sydney Smith, Sir G. Lewis, Whewell, Lord Kings-
down, Dean Milman, Senior, Eastlake, Hawtrey, &c.
To this list must now be added the name of Grote—our
latest loss, and lamented over by all who are capable of
appreciating great learning, a most upright intellect, and
a gentle and generous temper. The gaps thus made
have been well and honourably filled up and the fame
of the Club fully sustained. Yet, when looking round
our dinner-table, I cannot but feel at times how much
the individualities are changed since I first sat there !

* At this Centenary dinner, Lord Brougham, then in his 84th or 85th
year, was present : but unable to sit more than an hour at table.

With the exception of Lord Stanhope I am now the oldest member.

At one period, some years ago, we had a remarkable group of Homeric scholars in the Club, and frequent discussions of high interest arose out of their conjunction. When Grote, Gladstone, Macaulay, Milman, George Lewis, Mure, and Hawtrey came almost simultaneously on this field of old and various controversy, it could not happen but that there should be some keen conflict evolved. Scepticism and enthusiastic belief were both engaged, with sundry shades of opinion between. No subject more prolific of materials for learned dispute than the Homeric poems —none better fitted to adorn and reward the controversy. Macaulay's marvellous memory here came into full play, in aid of any opinions he espoused.

Another discussion of later date I am led to mention, because it was closed by a letter to me from Sir George Lewis, one of the last that learned man and upright statesman ever wrote. The dispute turned on human longevity, Macaulay and Lewis affirming their persuasion that no authentic record could be produced of life exceeding a hundred years. A Review I had formerly written of Flourens' work 'Sur la Longevité humaine,' brought me into the controversy; and I urged against them—successfully as I think—that in every age, country, and race of men, we had the concurrent record of ages much exceeding a hundred; and further, that the extreme diversities of human stature and weight are at least as great in proportion as these many alleged excesses of age—that the absence, in fact, of anomalous instances of the latter would be in itself a greater anomaly. It was easy to support this thesis, while admitting at the same time the great liability to error in all ordinary statements on the subject. In 1863, scarcely a fortnight before his death, I received a letter from Sir G. Lewis, admitting with his wonted candour that he had been wrong in his limit, an *authentic* case having just occurred to him of life prolonged to 103 years. I have myself since seen a person, still living, who numbers 106 years, well attested by documentary proof. The doctrine of Flourens, founded on a fanciful relation of the period of growth to the duration of life—that a hundred years is the normal life of man—carries its refutation on the face of it. But I see no just reason to doubt the affirmation and evidence, coming to us both from ancient and modern times, of numerous instances much more remarkable than those just named.*

Were I skilled in anecdote, which I am not, I might relate many other incidents and discussions occurring within my memory of the Club; all deriving interest from the intellectual character of the men concerned in them. Boswell, as is well known, was one of the earlier members, brought in under the skirts of men greater than himself. His notices of some of the dinners show that Dr. Johnson exercised there his wonted arbitrary sway in all conversation. The tortuous writing of

---

* The cases of Jenkins and the Countess of Desmond may be deemed apocryphal; but we cannot so easily put aside that of Thomas Parr, accredited by the celebrated Harvey, who examined his body after death.

Boswell's own name in one page of our earlier records, curiously shows him as even then addicted to that excess in wine which afterwards became habitual to him. Dr. Hawtrey at one time projected writing a history of the Club from its commencement; and probably would have done this, had his life been continued. The scheme may hereafter be renewed, though time is ever rendering such traditional history more vague.

Macaulay and Sydney Smith were the members last elected into the Club before the date of my own election. With the latter I was already connected by the closest family tie, that of my own marriage—with the former I became so afterwards by the marriage of my eldest Son. The peculiar faculties of these two remarkable men were never more strikingly displayed than at the dinners of the Club. The provocation to put forth wit, wisdom, and learning was felt and fully answered, and every dinner vivified by them. The joyous humour of Sydney Smith played over and lightened the more solid and copious learning of Macaulay. He was lost to us five years afterwards—a loss not to London society alone, but to the sound practical sense and conduct of English public life. Fourteen years later Lord Macaulay disappeared from among us—to me individually the loss of a friend, to whom, irrespectively of family ties, I had become more closely attached every year of life. His qualities and faculties of mind are fresh in the memory of so many that they need no commemoration here. He was devoted to the Club, and rarely absent from it. If redundant at times in speech and argument, this could hardly be deemed an usurpation, seeing how they were employed. If he ever seemed to trample upon an opponent, it was not from any will to do so, but simply from the overwhelming knowledge he brought to the combat. I well remember the blank that was felt by all at the first meeting of the Club after his death.

Hallam, not less constant in his presence there, died only a few months before Macaulay—a friend of forty years' standing, and endeared to me further by my attachment to his two remarkable sons, Arthur and Henry Hallam, prematurely and unhappily lost to him and to others. Though dying so young, they have left memories behind them, embalmed, as concerns Arthur, in some of the most beautiful poetry of our time.* From Vienna and Sienna severally, where their deaths occurred with but few years between, I received the most touching letters from Hallam himself, written on the very days of these great losses of his life. His own latter years were clouded by a paralytic seizure, which I mention only from the effect on him, rarely found in such cases, of diffusing a placid gentleness over the sterner qualities of his mind. He still indeed clung to society; but submitted patiently to the altered conditions of his appearance in it. A physician can best estimate the moral rectitude expressed in this gentle acquiescence,

---

* The volume entitled *In Memoriam*, by the Poet Laureate. I once spent a day with Arthur Hallam on the Lakes of Killarney. I had gone thither to see his father, whose health and spirits had been much affected by a ten weeks' confinement in a house on the Lower Lake, opposite the Isle of Innisfallen, where, by a fall from a rock, he had fractured his leg, and sustained other severe injury. It was pleasant to me to know that by this visit I gave aid towards his recovery.

supervening on a mind disputative and dogmatical in its natural bent.

It is not generally known that he refused a baronetcy, pressed upon him in the most flattering terms by Sir Robert Peel. He came to consult me on the subject, and, though reluctantly, I acquiesced in the reasons which led him finally to decline it. The statue of Hallam in St. Paul's strikingly pourtrays his massive intellectual features, and the general aspect of the man. In reference to this monument, I have pleasure in recollecting that, as one of a small committee (including among others Gladstone, Milman, Lord Houghton and Grote) to determine on the inscription, I aided in deciding the vote for an English instead of the Latin one originally proposed. Juvenal, when vindicating Latin itself against Greek, for Roman use, furnishes an apt argument for the decision in question.*

Lord Holland was a member of the Club when I became so, but died a few months afterwards. He too was a friend of thirty years' standing; endeared to me,

---

* The largest of Hallam's works, the 'History of the Literature of Europe in the .15th, 16th, and 17th centuries,' is that least known to the world. Replete with learning and just and eloquent criticism, it failed of the success of his earlier writings, from causes almost inevitable in its construction. The scheme of such a History, perhaps too large in itself, involved the necessity of choice among three methods, based severally on the divisions of time, of country, and of literary subject—all important, but each method more or less excluding the other two. Hallam more than once came to talk with me on the question before he began to write. The difficulty just stated was fully felt and discussed. Eventually he decided to take periods of time as the substratum of his work ; but the alterations he introduced in his progress show how much he was taxed by these conflicting plans of narrative.

as to all who knew him, by qualities in great part individual to himself, but in some sort hereditary in his family. The remarkable society and manner of life at Holland House have been often described, and by no one more vividly than Lord Macaulay, in one of his Essays taken from the ' Edinburgh Review.' I am not prone to extol the past at the expense of the present, but I nevertheless must state my feeling that nothing in London life has yet replaced what was the habitual society of Holland House. The London Season, as it is called, abounds in good dinners and good company; and these dinners take high rank among our social usages. But at Holland House (itself a classical spot) there met almost daily, during a series of years, round a luxurious table, guests eminent in such various ways, that their mere conjunction stamped its character on the society. English and Foreign Ministers and Diplomatists, men of learning and of science, historians, poets, artists and wits, were so skilfully commingled as to make it sure that none but a master-hand could have accomplished the result.

The master-hand here was that of the mistress, Lady Holland—a remarkable woman in every way, well-remembered by all who knew her—difficult to describe to those who did not. Supreme in her own mansion and family, she exercised a singular and seemingly capricious tyranny even over guests of the highest rank and position. Capricious it seemed, but there was in reality *intention* in all she did; and this intention was the maintenance of power, which she gained and strenuously used, though not without discretion in fixing its limits. No one knew better when to change her mood, and to soothe by kind and flattering words the provocation she had just given, and was very apt to give. In this latter case, indeed, she was aided by a native generosity of mind which never failed to show itself in kindness where kindness was wanted. In my long and intimate knowledge of Lady Holland, I never knew her desert an old friend, whatever his condition might be. Many things, seemingly wilful and incongruous in her, might be explained through this happier quality of mind blended with that love of power which, fostered by various circumstances, pervaded every part of her life. The influence she exercised was doubtless aided by large general reading, of which she made sedulous and skilful use. Her management of conversation at the dinner table—sometimes arbitrary and in rude arrest of others, sometimes courteously inviting the subject—furnished a study in itself. Every guest felt her presence, and generally more or less succumbed to it. She was acute in distinguishing between real and false merit, and merciless in her treatment of the latter. Not a woman of wit in words, she had what might well be called consummate practical wit in all her relations to society. Once only, and that very late in life, she spoke to me of the labour she underwent in maintaining the position thus acquired. The information was not necessary. My own observation had already made me well but silently aware of it.

My personal relations to Holland House, fostered by much previous intercourse in Italy, were of the most

agreeable kind from the beginning, and the lapse of
time in no way altered them.   Despite Lady Holland's
imperious rule in all matters of society, I was a guest
almost at my own bidding, and often passed the night
at this picturesque old mansion, abounding in so many
recollections of men and times.   My profession doubtless
served in some degree to maintain this intimacy.   My
politics, never much more than neutral, and rather tending to the other side, had certainly nothing to do with
it.   The political visitors of Holland House were of
course almost exclusively of the Whig party ; though it
was always matter of rejoicing to Lady Holland when
she could catch a stray Tory to mingle with them.*   But
political party was better leavened by the admixture of
literary men and eminent foreigners, who under her invitation found place at this table.   Lord Holland himself
came to it each day wholly ignorant whom he was to
find there ; but greeting all alike with his genial smile,
and animating all by the charm of his conversation, and
by a ·flow and felicity of anecdote peculiar to himself ;
the effect heightened by his own enjoyment of it.   He sat
always at a corner of the dinner-table, to which I doubt
whether he ever himself ventured to invite a guest.   The
writings he has left behind him give no just or adequate

* Mr. Gifford's wish was a very reasonable one, that they could ' get up
a Holland House on the Tory side of the question.'   Lady Holland seldom
failed in attaining an object she desired.   But this occurred in the case of
Lord Dudley, whom she vainly sought to obtain as a guest at Holland
House.   I rather think there had been some previous quarrel in Italy.   But
when I once accidentally asked Lord Dudley the reason, I recollect his
answer to have been, that ' he did not choose to be tyrannised over while
he was eating his dinner.'

idea of Lord Holland's abilities or of his admirable qualities in social life. They present that disparity which is often so strangely marked in faculties seemingly the closest in relation ; of which disparity his Uncle Mr. Fox was himself a remarkable instance. The tongue is often much more eloquent in style than the pen.*

I cannot attempt a list of the accustomed guests at Holland House during the days of its greatest renown. On the memory of the moment I may name, as those whom I most constantly saw there—Lord Grey, Lord Melbourne, Lord Lansdowne, Lord J. Russell, Lord Durham, Lord Brougham, Lord Palmerston, Lord Carlisle, Lord Althorp, Lord Lauderdale, Tierney, Mackintosh, Horner, Macaulay, Sydney Smith, Hallam, Rogers, Jekyll, Luttrell, Frere, Moore, Charles Ellis, &c. I am noting here a bygone generation, for only one of those I have named is now alive.

During the progress of the Reform Bill and the agitations attending it, the Holland House dinners were often a sort of miniature Cabinet, in the persons assembled and the matters discussed. A frequent guest at these dinners, I recollect one of them which ended to myself in a whimsical contrast. Called away hastily by a message from town, I quitted the table at which

---

* I have the picture still before me of Lord Holland lying tranquilly on his bed when attacked with gout—his admirable sister Miss Fox beside him, reading aloud, as she generally did on these occasions, some one of Miss Austen's novels, of which he was never wearied. I well recollect the time when these charming novels, fresh and almost unique in their style of humour, burst suddenly on the world. It was sad that their writer did not live to witness the growth of her fame.

were sitting several of the Ministers—the Premier Lord Grey amongst them—in earnest conversation on the progress of the Bill, then in one of its critical stages. A few minutes after, I got into an ill-lighted Kensington omnibus, in which I found half-a-dozen people loudly and passionately discussing the same subject, with those affirmations of 'certain knowledge' and 'the best authority,' so common in disputes of this nature, especially where little is really known. Sitting silently in a dark corner of the omnibus, I derived much amusement from this sudden change of place and company. It pictured whimsically the diversities, as well as resemblances, common to all grades of social and political life.

It had been often predicted that the society of Holland House would be wholly broken up by Lord Holland's death. It was not so. Though transferred for the most part to the town-house in South Street, and infringed upon by many other deaths, the singular talent of Lady Holland, aided by affection for his memory, kept together the habitual members of this society as long as she herself lived. Her dinners were still amongst the most agreeable in London. I well remember one in October 1845—the last she ever gave —when Thiers and Lord Palmerston met, as I believe, for the first time, smothering at the table the angry feelings of prior diplomacy. At this dinner I distinctly perceived, though to others less intimate they might not have been obvious, the first signs of that illness which closed Lady Holland's life less than a month afterwards.

I have said more of her than I intended ; but the interest I feel in her memory is one appertaining to a long period of my own life.

I cannot quit the subject of Holland House, without mentioning one who was a member of the family for forty years, and had acquired much influence in it. This was Mr. Allen—familiarly called John Allen—a man of encyclopædic literature, of hard unflinching Whig politics, and a temperament of general scepticism ; yet with sundry warm affections lying underneath. He was cast in a strong Scotch mould both of mind and body—the former nurtured by constant reading and excellent society, the latter pampered by daily luxurious dinners throughout the year. Sitting always at the bottom of the table, before carving had been transferred to the sideboard, he yet mixed largely in the conversation as an expounder of facts, and a sharp commentator on the words and opinions of others. Even Lady Holland, who found pleasure in exciting him, did not escape his angry contradictions and had a certain dim fear of them. Without native wit himself, he had learnt to appreciate it by living so long among the choicest wits of the day. To many Parliamentary orators he furnished the rough material which they refined into eloquence. In the well-known engraving of the Library at Holland House, his figure is well delineated ; as is also that of the librarian-page, a subordinate but singular member of the household, who knew more about books than many men of literary name.

The elder brother of Sydney Smith (called Bobus by his friends, though his noble and somewhat stern countenance seemed to repel the familiarity) was seen now and then at Holland House, but rarely in any other society. Connected with him by close personal friendship as well as by family ties, I have some claim to speak of this remarkable man, the most accomplished scholar and the most profound thinker I have ever known. Gifted with the power of putting his thoughts into eloquent and forcible speech, he added to this a rich adornment of wit ; sparingly employed indeed, and more in the sharp sarcastic vein of Talleyrand than with the joyous redundance of his brother's humour. An argument—metaphysical, moral, or literary—with Robert Smith was a strong intellectual exercise to his opponent, a luxury to any intelligent listener. I mention these things because his habits of life prevented their being known beyond a limited circle of friends. He was perhaps too sternly a despiser of the world around him— happier with his Homer, Æschylus, Lucretius, and Dante, than in any other society. He could better indeed talk with and amuse children than mingle with common men, of which his relations to my own children gave me frequent and pleasant proof. The excellence of his Latin versification is well known to Eton scholars ; and the Lucretian poems, republished by his son Lord Lyveden, attest his love for this the noblest of the Latin poets. His recitation of favourite passages from the great authors I have just named, had a grandeur of voice and emphasis which gave fresh grandeur to the passages themselves. It was Lord Dudley, I believe, who, being called upon in a classical discussion for his opinion on the relative excellencies of the several Roman poets, named Lucretius, Catullus, and Bobus, as taking first rank among them, passing on without stop to Virgil, Horace, Juvenal, &c.

Mr. Smith and his brother Sydney died within little more than a fortnight of each other, and of similar organic disease of the heart. I was present at the very touching scene of their last meeting, with the event in view to both. I have before me some beautiful and touching lines written by the former shortly before his death, and, as they show, in immediate anticipation of it. These I willingly subjoin. They epitomise in fact the sentiment of his life.*

---

* ' Hic jacet '—O humanarum meta ultima rerum,
    Ultra quam labor et luctus curæque quiescunt ;
    Ultra quam pendentur opes et gloria flocci
    Et redit ad nihilum vana hæc et turbida vita.
    Ut te respicerent homines ! quæ bella per orbem,
    Qui motus animorum, et quanta pericula nostra
    Acciperent facilem sine cæde et sanguine finem !
    Tu mihi versare ante oculos—non tristis imago,
    Sed monitrix ut me ipse regam, domus hæc mihi cum sit
    Vestibulum tumuli, et senii penultima sedes. *February* 1845.

CHAPTER IX.

PURSUING my narrative in the same desultory way, I may mention that it was at Holland House I made the acquaintance of Sir Philip Francis; whom, by his invitation, I afterwards occasionally visited at his house in St. James's Square. At that time the suspicion of his being Junius had not reached the degree of assurance which the acute argument of Macaulay afterwards gave to it; suggesting, if not warranting, the declaration of a great lawyer that a man might be hung on less evidence. Some years afterwards, Mr. Woodfall, the representative of that publisher whose name comes to us in connection with the ' Letters of Junius,' met Macaulay at my breakfast-table; bringing with him in a box all the original manuscripts of these famous letters, which have subserved to so much controversy—involving, I believe, more than twenty names of alleged authorship. I never heard the question mooted in Sir Philip Francis's presence; nor can I contribute more towards its solution.than by saying that his temperament, even thus late in life, was of the *Junius stamp ;* and that I never knew a man more likely to persist obstinately and angrily in a denial he had once given, irrespectively of other more special motives for concealment.

The Junius controversy has had, I think, four or five distinct revivals within my time, besides much scattered conjecture in the intervals between. Never was a subject better fitted in all its details to excite and keep up controversy. It is in truth not ãmiss to have questions of this harmless kind pending from one generation to another. They agreeably diversify the turmoils of political and social life.*

I saw much of Horner, both at Holland House and elsewhere, and felt the esteem common to all who knew him, for his fine intellectual and moral qualities seldom so happily combined. I witnessed the earlier appearances of that malady which prematurely closed his life. He had been contemporary with Brougham in Edinburgh education, and in advent on the field of political life. If the genius of the former was more ardent and subtle, the moral quality of Horner's intellect was of higher stamp and more entire consistency. Had he possessed even in part the strong physical temperament of Lord Brougham, he would, I believe, have reached higher fame as a statesman than the latter, and left more enduring marks of his career.

Lord Lauderdale was among the most assiduous frequenters of Holland House, and always welcome to Lady Holland, notwithstanding his political economy,

---

* The latest of these Junius *paroxysms* is that evoked by the remarkable volume of Mr. Twistleton, in which the redundance of the evidence may almost be said to impair its effects. Mr. Hayward is by far the ablest of those writers who deny the authorship of Francis. His essay on the subject a few years ago was remarkable for its power of close and ingenious scrutinv

which she abhorred, and a racy dialect of Lothian Scotch, which sounded somewhat incongruously at her table. He was a man of hard unflinching common sense, and a certain coarse shrewdness, which rendered him very useful in the management of party politics in Scotland. His activity vented itself in another way, less suited it might seem to his temperament. If a family *imbroglio* occurred, whatever its nature, in the large circle in which Lord Lauderdale lived, he was sure to be found in the midst of it, as adviser, mediator, or controller. I never knew him more alert and happy than when he had a matter of this kind in hand. He was the most inveterate snuff-taker I ever knew, and learned in this luxury. Each one of his numerous canisters had some history or date inscribed on it, and even his bed betokened his frequent recourse to them.

I have already spoken of my intimate friendship with Macaulay and Hallam. To these names I willingly add those of Mackintosh and Whewell. Though dating from a different time, my intimacy with those two remarkable men was close and unbroken to the end of their lives. I had seen Sir J. Mackintosh before he went to India. After his return, I knew him both as friend and physician; and saw him very continually both at his own house, and in the various society which he loved and adorned. His character, intellectual and moral, was well deserving study. It has been admirably drawn by Macaulay in one of his Reviews, and brought into striking comparison and contrast with that of

Hallam. Argument, logically framed and learnedly illustrated, but ever on his part candid and without passion, was the great luxury of Mackintosh's life—a luxury not less to anyone who heard him engaged with a combatant worthy of himself. But unlike many of the men I have just named, he was tolerant even of mediocrity, if affording him in any way exercise for his reasoning powers. His learning and logic, if not appreciated by others, reacted pleasurably upon himself. I have elsewhere spoken of his conversational conflicts with Madame de Staël. Metaphysical and literary questions were those in which he had greatest delight; and in his devotion to them, he too often put aside that steady labour which might have gained him one of the highest places among English historians. Many passages in his Journals show, even painfully, his earnest longing to accomplish objects which his habits of life rendered unattainable.

In the 'Memoir of Sir J. Mackintosh's Life,' by his Son, there are three communications of great interest, from Scarlett, Sydney Smith, and Jeffrey—each memoir illustrating in a different way the character of Mackintosh, and thus becoming characteristic of the writer himself. To these, at the request of his Son, I added a fourth, having reference to the views of Mackintosh on the question of a ' moral faculty ' in Man, as they are given in his 'Dissertation on the Progress of Ethical Philosophy.' It was some sanction to my writing on the subject, that he had placed this treatise in my hands before its publication, and that we had often discussed together the many knotty questions it involves.

My friendship with Whewell was one of thirty-five years. Our intercourse was chiefly in London; but my family and I paid him occasional visits at Trinity Lodge. I saw and corresponded much with him while he was printing his two works (which might better have been embodied into one) on the Inductive Sciences. Of the latter of these works most of the proof sheets were sent me for revision ; but it was at the busiest period of my practice, and I had hard work to keep up with the rate of printing, prompted by his ardour of action in everything he undertook. At that time the mind of Whewell worked with a sort of gigantic impulse upon each of the many subjects—perhaps too many— to which it addressed itself. On the fate of his singular anonymous work, the 'Plurality of Worlds,' he hung with a sort of impatient interest. A few days before its publication he sent me a copy, with a letter purporting that the author, a friend of his, wished to have my opinion on the hypothesis propounded. Though suspecting the real authorship, I took advantage of this anonymous request to send back a somewhat free criticism upon it. It was easy to praise the great ability and ingenuity of the work, while rejecting a conclusion defensible chiefly, if not solely, from the impossibility of ever *proving* the contrary. Sir D. Brewster, whom I frequently saw at this time, wrote a hasty and somewhat petulant answer to Whewell, but the controversy went little further, tempting though the question is to human speculation.*

I am carrying on my narrative with so little regard to dates, that I may mention here two other men, of whom I saw much in society during the earlier period of my London life. These were Malthus and Ricardo— names belonging to the history of that time, and deriving their reputation from very similar sources : one of them, the austere socialist philosopher as he was deemed, and, as respects Man at least, the precursor of Darwin in the doctrine of what has been called the ' struggle for life ; '—the other, Ricardo, a hard political economist, or then regarded as such ; but who, in reviving and applying the doctrines of Adam Smith, paved the way to some of the most beneficial acts of modern legislation. His benignity of character and simple but earnest manner in argument often made converts where his books had failed to do so.

The personal aspect of Malthus, to those who had known him only through the ' Essay on Population ' (a book however more railed at than read), generally excited some surprise. With genial, even gentle expression of features, he had a tremulous stammering voice,

---

* Had Whewell been yet living he would have rejoiced in the presumption derived from recent spectroscopic observations, that many at least of the Nebulæ (*stardust* as he contemptuously called them) are really nebulous or gaseous in their nature, and not groups of worlds deriving this aspect from their immensity of distance in space. But other recent discoveries, identifying many of the material constituents of the sun and stars with those of our globe, have much more direct bearing against his hypothesis. The theological element of the question may rightly be removed altogether.

seemingly little fitted for the utterance of any doctrine which could be deemed dangerous to social welfare. The present state of the world has sanctioned many opinions of Malthus which during his lifetime were angrily contradicted. Nor have we yet reached all the contingencies inevitably besetting the human race, to which his doctrines directly apply.

In connection with the same period of my London life, I may mention the name of Mr. Scarlett (Lord Abinger), who, notwithstanding his then unexampled success at the Bar, lived much in society and was ever well marked when present in it. I knew him long as a friend ; later in life professionally. With much various knowledge and great conversational faculty, his forensic habits and success were sometimes too apparent in his demeanour at the dinner-table. The control he had obtained in the Courts he could not relinquish out of them. Confident in his argumentative power he loved by contradiction to provoke it ; and whatever the subject might be, rarely conceded a point to his adversary. I have heard Sydney Smith say, that he believed the most flattering compliment Scarlett ever uttered was one addressed to himself, in the course of an argument between them : ' Do you know, Sydney, you're not altogether in the wrong.' The anecdote is thoroughly illustrative of the man. His florid and genial countenance sometimes entrapped strangers into disputes, which would have been shunned had their opponent been recognised and better understood. The power he exercised over juries was a wonderful one ; but the long use of this faculty was thought to have somewhat impaired his excellence as a judge. I have often heard Lord Abinger describe, with much amusing illustration, some of the methods he employed, as a barrister, to win over a jury. One of these consisted in closely scrutinising, while the trial was proceeding, the aspects of the twelve men in the jury-box. If discovering, as could often be done, that some one of them was distinctly superior to the rest in intelligence and other qualities which influence common men—to this person, when addressing the jury, he especially directed his eye and speech, winning the good-will of the flattered juryman, and through him the verdict sought for.

Though less familiarly known in general society than many of the eminent men of whom I have spoken, the grave and dignified presence of Sir Samuel Romilly, and his striking intellectual expression, marked him in every company in which he was seen. Without pretending to define exactly what is meant by a ' Roman countenance,' I would say that his well realised the common understanding of the phrase. His private writings, as we find them embodied in the Memoirs of his Life, give ample evidence of the high principles and pure affections associated with this outward demeanour, and in no way tainted by the successes of his professional career. His manner of death gave painful proof of the depth of these affections.

In singular contrast to Sir S. Romilly came Lord Erskine; of whom indeed I saw much less, and at a time when his faculties had undergone a decay more

obvious to others than to himself. He was still eager
and eloquent in speech; but with a certain restless irritability, augmented, as I believe, by narrow worldly
circumstances, and by what he deemed the neglect of
his former political friends. His mind too, when I knew
him, was clouded by little foibles and superstitions. I
well recollect a dinner at Sir S. Romilly's, where his
agitation was curiously shown in his reluctance to sit
down as one of thirteen at table, and by the relief he
expressed when the fourteenth guest came in. His life
had been one of *meteoric* kind throughout, vanishing in
mist as such lives are prone to do.

A second striking contrast to Romilly was presented
by another Equity Judge of this time, Sir John Leach;
familiarly known to me both at his own house and in
that general society which he assiduously frequented.
His was a character made up of curious contrasts. As
a Judge (I speak here from general report of the time)
he was able and energetic; but irritable and impatient
in his self-will, and often very offensive in his Court. In
society he was a petit-maître in dress and demeanour ; his
manner obsequious and fawning ; his conversation made
up of platitudes and commonplaces. Out of his profession indeed Leach was an ignorant man ; and his
Continental tours, methodised strictly for every day
before he set out, did little to redeem this ignorance. I
once accidentally fell in with him in one of these journeys,
and was much amused by his technical rule of travel,
little guided by any knowledge of the places he visited.
There were then no Handbooks from which to gather

ready-made knowledge, and I recollect one conversation with him after a German tour, in which, while
speaking with admiration of Prague, he led me clearly
to infer that he had never heard of this City before.
I may notice, and with some belief in its truth, the
opinion that it was the influence of Sir John Leach with
George IV., and the advice he gave, which determined
the trial of Queen Caroline, despite the opinions of
Lord Liverpool and his colleagues in opposition to it.

While thus briefly noting some of the eminent men of
the last generation with whom it has been my fortune
to become connected, I may shortly notice also the
many remarkable women whom I have attended as
patients and known as friends. I have already spoken
of Lady Holland, Princess Lieven, Madame de Staël,
Miss Edgeworth, Lady Davy, and others. From my
memory while writing I may further name Mrs. Somerville, Mrs. Marcet, Joanna Baillie, Lady Anne Lindsay,
Lady Dacre, Lady Morley, Lady Blessington, Mrs.
Siddons, the Misses Berry, Mrs. Barbauld, Mrs. Fry,
Mrs. Piozzi, &c. And to these I would fain add the
less familiar name of Lydia White, cherished in the
recollections of those, now very few indeed, who still
survive her. This lively and kind-hearted woman, with
no pretence to learning of any kind, and suffering under
a disease of which she well knew the certain and fatal
issue, yet almost to the last made her house in Park
Street the open and welcome resort of the best literary
society of the day. Dinner parties elsewhere sent their
most approved guests to 'look in at Lydia's' in the

evening, where all who came were sure of a genial reception, of good society, and thorough freedom from constraint. The whimsical licence of her own speech gave some sanction to it in her guests. Many circles of society have gained fame in memoirs of the time, though less deserving it than the pleasant, open-hearted evenings at Lydia White's.

I have just named Mrs. Marcet, whom I knew both as friend and physician, to the end of her life. Her works well denote her vigorous understanding and various and accurate knowledge, sustained by constant intercourse with the first scientific men of her day. It is no slight eulogium to say that Faraday derived his first aspirations after Chemistry from one of her volumes; and that the acknowledgment of this is found in letters where he signs himself her ‘affectionate pupil’—an expression equally honourable to both.

Of Joanna Baillie too I saw much both as a friend and patient. Her gentle simplicity, with a Scotch tinge colouring it to the end of life, won the admiration even of those who knew nothing of her power of dramatic poetry. It was pleasant to visit her in the quiet house at Hampstead, in which she lived with her sister Agnes. She reached, I think, her ninety-second year. Agnes lived to a hundred. Their brother, Dr. Baillie, exhausted by years of professional toil, when youth was already gone by, and reaching repose only when it was too late to be of avail, died when but sixty-four. He was the physician with whom I was most intimate in my early professional life—a man of simple and generous nature, in no way sullied by his large intercourse with the world.

From my long intimacy with them I might have spoken here of Miss Berry and her sister, whose house and hospitality kept together, even to the extreme old age of these ladies, one of the most agreeable circles in London ; associating old times with the new, and bringing personal recollections of Horace Walpole into conjunction with the people and habits of the present day. But the ample 'Memoir of Miss Berry' by Lady Theresa Lewis, lately published, makes this needless. I attended both sisters to the hour of their death. The Queen invited Miss Berry to a private interview when in her ninetieth year. This act of kindness was deeply felt.

Though Mrs. Somerville is yet living, and therefore not within the scope I have assigned to my narrative, I cannot forbear saying a few words about this remarkable woman ; sanctioned by a friendship of fifty years, and by the fact that her long absence from England has left to a few only the recollection of those other qualities and accomplishments which would have signalised her, apart even from her mathematical and other scientific attainments. A stranger might have sat by Mrs. Somerville at table, and admired her gentle and pleasing conversation, without a suspicion that she had rendered into English the ' Mécanique Céleste' of Laplace, and written the best book we possess on the ' Connection of the Physical Sciences.' I venture to claim for myself a slight merit in relation to the latter work. When she explained to me the first outline of her plan, limited to

the connection of Astronomy with Optics and the phenomena of light, I suggested—holding in view the more
general connection of all the physical sciences—that she
should extend her scheme to the form in which the work
now appears, and the suggestion, seconded by her own
judgment, was adopted. The value of the volume is
well attested by the numerous editions it has gone
through, each one corrected up to the latest dates of
scientific discovery. I brought the proof sheets of the
ninth edition with me from Florence to London, for
revision on the road, but could find very little to add
or alter in them.

Some years before, knowing that she wished it, I
wrote for the 'Quarterly Review' an article on her two
volumes of 'Physical Geography'—an easy task where
there was so much to praise. Less ambitious in title
and form than the 'Cosmos' of Humboldt, the works of
Mrs. Somerville embrace really the whole scope of his
design, and, as I think, with a more lucid definition and
arrangement of the subjects it includes. Her latest work
is that on Molecular Science, published when she had
reached her eighty-eighth year.

The mention of Humboldt's name reminds me that I
have not spoken of him among the men of mark with
whom I have chanced to come into relation. I frequently met him both in England and abroad ; and
once, in 1840, passed an interesting day at his villa in
the gardens of Sans-Souci at Potsdam. I recollect this
visit more especially from the incident of my being presented by Humboldt to the late King of Prussia, whom

we met walking in the gardens. He was accompanied by Prince John of Saxony and his sister the Princess Amelia—the former a vigorous translator of Dante into German verse; the latter the authoress of several volumes of German dramas of social life, which 1 read to the present day with unabated pleasure. With these Royal personages and Humboldt, I walked for some time in the gardens under the light of a beautiful autumnal evening—one of the agreeable accidents of travel not to be forgotten. No presentation at a levee or drawing-room could have left equal mark on the memory.

The diversely-composed character of the late King of Prussia has now become matter of history; and this interview of half an hour does not enable me to add anything to the estimate of it. What I may venture to affirm is that the events of 1865 and 1870 would not have occurred had he been still on the throne. Prince John's literary and scientific tastes gave him large part in the conversation at Sans-Souci ; and he put many questions to me touching my travels in Iceland, of which Humboldt had spoken to him. Little anticipation existed at that time of the changes which have placed this Prince (now King of Saxony) in such altered and unwonted relations to the Prussian monarchy ! Germany has been living a century within the years just elapsed. If the future were ever to be reached by human prediction, the establishment of the unity of this great people might be cited as an event of happiest augury for Europe in all time to come.

Some years after this visit to Potsdam I wrote for the 'Quarterly Review' an article on the second and third volumes of Humboldt's 'Cosmos;' in which I commented with some freedom, but I think with justice, on the outline and method of execution of the work—one too large to be executed by a single hand, however powerful its grasp. I heard with more regret than surprise that he had been offended by the criticism, while ignorant of its author. The homage paid to him during a long series of years rendered him singularly susceptible to all that touched on his fame; and the reception by the world of what he considered his crowning work was not such as to fulfil the expectations he had formed. He had obviously never satisfied himself with his own definition of 'Cosmos;' and was the more sensitive to critical comment on the undertaking which he had thus too ambitiously designated. I slightly knew his brother Wilhelm Humboldt; a man inferior in all that concerned the physical sciences, but, as I venture from his writings to think, of larger philosophy and a higher moral temperament. The posthumous fame of Alexander Humboldt, prejudiced by the unwarrantable publication of his letters, has scarcely equalled that which he maintained while alive. But he must ever be remembered as the man whose researches and writings have raised Physical Geography to the rank of a science, and furnished its most admirable illustrations.

The same visit to Berlin gave me the opportunity of passing some time with Ehrenberg (then the *master-eye* in Infusorial research), and of inspecting through his microscopes some of the extraordinary discoveries made in what he has himself not inaptly termed '*the milky way of the smallest organisation.*' It is in this 'milky way,' that science, aided by still more perfect instruments, has since obtained such wonderful knowledge of the intimate parts of living organisation, under the endless forms they assume in the natural world.   I have had, subsequently to this meeting at Berlin, various communications from Ehrenberg ; one of them, in 1848, including specimens of that strange *bread-mould* of bright vermilion colour (containing two microscopic fungi and one animal organism) which on a particular day appeared in Berlin, tainting the bread and other farinaceous matters in different parts of the City.   The Asiatic cholera was prevailing there at the time ; and, naturally enough, many were disposed to connect this phenomenon with the presence of the epidemic.   Such conclusion might seem almost justified by a similar appearance of *red mould* on bread, occurring in Philadelphia in 1832 when the Cholera was prevailing in that city.*   It is, however, clearly inadmissible, seeing that these are single and exceptional cases amidst the endless number of examples which the history of Cholera has brought before us.   But still I may remark that the facts just

---

* The records by ancient historians of *showers of blood*, are doubtless referrible to the same physical cause as that denoted by the observations of Ehrenberg.   And we may thus more distinctly explain the story given by Quintus Curtius, of a *blood-rain* near the end of the siege of Tyre by Alexander ; – staining the bread of the Macedonian soldiers as well as of the besieged Tyrians, but frightening the latter into surrender.

noted come within that *class of phenomena* to which, in my opinion, we must look for explanation of the real origin of this disease—a subject to which I shall advert in a later page of this volume.

To the names of these great German naturalists, I may add that of another German, eminent in a very different way, whom at one time I met occasionally. This was Augustus Schlegel, a man well deserving credit in England from his ardent devotion to the greatest of our authors. His critical analysis of the plays of Shakespeare, in the ' Littérature Dramatique,' merges in the more wonderful translation which, in conjunction with Tieck, he accomplished of their total number. It was affirmed, I think by Klopstock, that if the text of the ' Iliad ' were lost, it might be well-nigh restored by Greek scholars from German versions of Homer. The same cannot be said of Shakespeare ; but it must be admitted that the translation is throughout one of wonderful vigour and ability, surmounting difficulties that might well be deemed insuperable, and meeting fully the requirement of Dryden that ' a translator should perfectly understand his author's tongue, and absolutely command his own.' It was amusing to listen to the sarcastic scorn—not wholly undeserved — with which Schlegel treated most of the English commentators on Shakespeare. ' To understand Shakespeare well, an Englishman must come to Germany,' was an expression I heard him use one day at Sir J. Mackintosh's dinner-table ; and it passed without contradiction. I have myself seen ' Romeo and Juliet ' acted at Dresden, with an excellence hardly to be surpassed. The subordinate parts, so often neglected on the English stage, were brought out with the care and completeness which they require and so amply repay.

I think it was at this dinner that I put a question to Schlegel, whether in his close reading and translating of Shakespeare, he had discovered any principle or plan upon which the transition was made, in the dialogue of the plays, from prose to verse, or from blank verse to rhyme ? If I am right in my memory of a conversation thus remote in time, he admitted that he had found no such rule or design. My own reading of Shakespeare with explicit reference to this question, while showing that such changes of style were often made in relation to the subject involved, or to give point to the close of a scene or speech, yet has furnished me with no clue whatever to anything like uniformity of purpose. The sole explanation of incongruities in Shakespeare is to be found, I believe, in that *sublime carelessness* which is characteristic of the genius of this wonderful man. Indifferent to common fame, he disdained the methods by which inferior authors strive to obtain it. But though unable myself to obtain a solution of the question just stated, I would suggest it to other readers as one of the many curious· problems which Shakespeare has bequeathed to us.*

* This allusion to Shakespeare tempts me into another anecdote, in which I had some concern. At a dinner now long ago, Lord Nugent (the greatest Shakespearian scholar of his day) affirmed that there was not, in the whole series of the plays, a single passage commending, directly or indirectly, the *moral qualities* of the dog. Thinking this to be impossible,

Among the remarkable foreigners whom I have known, I may briefly mention two singular persons, who some twenty-five or thirty years ago attracted a certain attention in England. These were Ugo Foscolo and Blanco White—men who might well have been born in different planets. Foscolo, full of genius and original thought as his writings show, was fiery and impulsive almost to the verge of madness. I have seen him, under the excitement of contradiction, rise from a dinner-table and stamp round the room, his knife in his hand. His declamation of Dante was almost terrific in effect. He seemed to revel in the horrors of the *Dolente regno*, of which his harsh voice intensified the description. He lived in the literary world for a time, and partially supported himself by his writings ; but, as might be expected, dropt gradually out of society and died in obscurity and neglect.

I accepted a wager which Lord Nugent offered me on the subject, with the concession of a year to make my research. Even with the aid of several friends, I failed to find any such passage ; and at the end of the year I paid the guinea I had lost. At a dinner at the Bishop of Exeter's, some time afterwards, where I related the anecdote, Mr. Croker with his wonted ingenuity struck upon a passage which came nearest perhaps to the point ; but it was an ingenious inference only, and would not have won me my wager.

Touching on Shakespeare, it is difficult to quit the subject. A year or two ago, at a dinner at my house, the question was started—which of the characters in all his plays most strikingly betokened the genius of the author? I ventured to bring forward Cleopatra ; seeing as I do in this wonderful portraiture not merely grandeur of conception, but with this a marvellous elaboration of all those details which colour and complete the picture. A friend of mine, of highest political position and alike eminent in literature, was present and took active part in the discussion; not concurring at the time, but promising fresh study of the play. Some time after, in sequel to this study, I obtained from him if not an entire acquiescence at least an expression of admiration equal to my own for the Cleopatra of Shakespeare.

I did all I could do to aid and solace him under his
decay, but his pride made even this a matter of difficulty.
The person whom I recollect as most resembling him
was his countryman, Fuseli ; as passionately eccentric in
social life as he was in his paintings,—a temperament
which clung to him, as I myself witnessed, to the hour
of his death. I cannot easily forget the benevolent
care with which Sir Thomas Lawrence watched over
Fuseli during the long illness thus ending.

Blanco White—half English half Spanish by descent
—was one of the most striking cases I have known of
' that painful thinking which corrodes the clay.' He lived
in an atmosphere of doubts and gloomy thoughts, all
directed to religious questions and the destinies of man.
His writings and the acts of his life show, what his
countenance and conversation well depictured, the unceasing and painful restlessness of his mind on these
topics. He sent for me frequently ; but the inborn
temperament of the man was too strong to allow of
remedy, and any relief I could give was speedily lost in
the chaos of changeful thoughts and speculations, which
haunted him to the hour of his death. The persistent
kindness of Archbishop Whately to Blanco White, in
spite of some obloquy incurred thereby, was one of the
many traits which do honour to the memory of that
excellent but eccentric prelate.

These brief notices of two men who struggled *alone*
in the stream of life, show, though very faintly, what are
the frequent experiences of the London physician ; and
show moreover the fitness of abstaining generally from

whatever might become a record of such anomalies in human character, where others besides the individuals themselves are affected by their delineation. Ugo Foscolo and Blanco White died leaving no near kindred behind them. Italy however has recently honoured the genius and literary labours of the former, by claiming his remains. Removed from Chiswick where he was buried, they are transferred to the Church of Santa Croce at Florence,—the city being illuminated on the occasion of this second and more solemn interment.

CHAPTER X.

THESE slight and scattered notices of the society in which I have passed much of my life might of course be largely extended, even limiting them as I have done to a generation now nearly gone by. A London physician has necessarily connection also with other circles of society less marked to the public eye, though all filling their several parts in the great drama of life. But of these I must speak only generally ; and the rather so as my intercourse with them has been more exclusively of professional or casual kind, and less intimate than with the society to which I have already alluded, where friendship was so often blended with professional relations.

I have often put to myself a question, which indeed every existing generation has motive and right to ask, as to its relations of *better* or *worse*—morally, intellectually, and socially—to the generation going before it. The question is one not readily answered. Even limiting it to social life and to that of London only, I find much difficulty in comparing what I now see around me with that which I saw and lived amidst, when first entering on the London world. The word *society* itself is not easy of definition, and is very variously interpreted by the

S

different circles composing it.   The changes which have
occurred, whatever their nature, have come on gradually;
and the estimate of them depends on the temperament
and changing moods of those who adventure opinions on
the subject.   That there is a certain balance of gain and
loss is a safe conclusion, but a very useless one, unless
expressed by details which few can render impartially
even to themselves.

Treating the matter very generally, I may say that
the changes which have occurred in my time, and especially those of *deterioration*, are chiefly such as result
from the *over-crowding* of the London world—a phrase
which will be appreciated by all who have lived in its
midst.   It is in truth a theme on which much might be
written, prospectively as well as for the present time ;
and nowhere with wider application than to our own
overgrown metropolis.   The rapid increase of numbers
in London is sufficiently shown by the decennial census.
The influence of this increase pervades the whole economy of social life from the highest to the lowest.   It
is testified generally by a more miscellaneous intermingling of the different elements of society—the lower
gaining, I fear it must be admitted, in their proportion
to the higher.   The crowded dinner-tables of the present
day, and still more those evening assemblages under
whatever fanciful name convoked—stifling breath as
well as conversation—have largely swelled society, but
not improved it.   The practical definition of a crowd, of
whatever rank it be composed, approaches closely to
that of a mob ; the intellect and happier refinements of

society alike suffer from it. The men of genius, literature and wit, are doubtless as numerous in London as
heretofore; but they are less marked individually in the
multitude, and many of them partially concealed by
their connection with the anonymous periodical writings
of the day.

I might enumerate, from my experience, other and more
important influences, moral as well as physical, of this
over-crowded life, were these things not alien to the
purpose of my narrative. There is however one particular result on which I would say a few words, inasmuch
as its effects upon society are patent to daily experience,
and call strongly for correction. This is the present
extravagant multiplication of societies and institutions
of every kind, dividing and subdividing all the concerns
of human life ; — charities, literature, science, art, the
professions, trades, and social intercourse in all its
shapes. Scheme follows scheme in rapid succession,
and the devising and prosecution of these schemes has
become itself a profession to many. With every allowance for increasing population and wealth, life and estate
in London are grievously over-ridden by the multitude
of the exactions thus imposed ; often wholly fruitless for
the objects assigned, and consuming in their method of
use the means that have been evoked for more laudable
purposes. Of the endless institutions thus created by
public charity, fashion, or credulity, many speedily
become mendicant ; while those of higher and better
purpose are starved in the struggle of competition. To
annul some of these institutions altogether, and to

concentrate others into co-operation, may be a work of difficulty, but is well deserving a vigorous effort to accomplish it. Those belonging to charitable objects especially need revision and reformation. I cannot doubt, from what I have myself seen, that the pauperism of London is augmented rather than relieved by their multiplicity and maladministration.

The classical scholar, designated as such, is, I think, not held in the same estimation as he was fifty or sixty years ago ; and this opinion I give, despite the numerous translations of Homer and others of the ancient poets, which have recently appeared in active competition of method and metre. Translations in verse do not always presume minute critical knowledge, and probably would be worse if fashioned upon it. From various causes scholars of the Bentley and Markland stamp are not likely to be as numerous as heretofore, or equally prized in the world. Perhaps, too, there is less familiarity now with our own great classics, save fragmentally through those multitudinous ephemeral writings which, while spreading knowledge over a larger surface, tend to make it more vague and fleeting. Even the ' Paradise Lost ' and Dryden's 'Fables' and Political Poems are now rather names than realities to the great mass of English readers. A stray line here and there, apt for quotation, represents pretty fairly the part they fill in the common literary knowledge or talk of the day.

The vast amount of talent and wit expended in periodical literature under different forms, is another notable characteristic of the times, influencing those who write, and those who read what is written. The seductions of a literature made thus facile of access, are not easily resisted. In effect of these and other causes, there is more general reading, but less of earnest individual study than formerly. The mere outward forms of folio and quarto exercised indeed a sort of compulsion over the student, who could not easily fling them aside as he does the light and loosely-bound volumes of modern literature; and who had no summary at hand, in Review or Magazine, to fill up the gaps in his own knowledge.

A few words more as to this periodical literature, so profusely augmented in quantity and power. The amount of anonymous writing appearing in this form is in truth one of the greatest marvels of the age;—writing often admirable in kind, and dealing with subjects of highest import to social and political life. The leading articles of the daily newspaper, upon which we cast a careless eye at the breakfast-table, had they been rooted out from the records of the last century, might justly have excited our admiration. Yet all this work of intellect is without name and ephemeral. It dies with the day that gave it birth—evoked again, if ever, only to prove the consistency or inconsistency of the later opinions put forth.

It is impossible not to regard this as a striking feature of the time in which we are living. The writing just described pervades English social life even to its lowest grades—happily tempered by knowledge, good taste,

and right temper in most instances, but capable of being
mischievously used—and too frequently so used—among
those with whom these qualities have little or no value
I have now and then looked back, and always with much
interest, at the newspapers of my early youth. Few
in number, tardy and limited in their circulation, scanty
of intelligence, and rarely and feebly touching on those
great questions which agitate the world, they were comparatively powerless for good or for evil. The modern
newspaper press holds this power in both ways; and holds
it at a time pregnant with changes of which it is at once
the interpreter and the agent. There is nothing new in
these comments. They must occur, more or less, to every
one who can observe and reason upon what they see
around them. If speaking on the subject here, it is
because I often and strongly feel the deep import of
these things to the welfare of the world—the *New World*
it may rightly be called, on this side the Atlantic as well
as on the other.

The large extension of physical science in all its
branches has not been without influence, even on the
literary society of the day. The numerous attempts to
popularise it are ever indeed left behind by its unceasing
progress ; and much illegitimate science has grown out
of the effort to reconcile its results with old opinions,
or with the fanciful theories and delusions periodically
arising in the world. But still the general increase of
physical knowledge may be said to have brought a new
and valuable element into the ordinary intercourse of

life. Few may know, or care to know, the particular metals and gases discovered in the Solar envelope ; but it is profitable even simply to understand that there are material elements in the Sun, Planets, and fixed Stars, identical with those most familiar to us on earth. And the effect of knowledge of this kind must be progressive, since science is ever advancing, while other learning lingers behind—investing itself in new contexture of words, or finding at intervals new channels and modes of development, but in its material essentially the same from one generation to another.

I may notice two other results, at first sight seemingly incongruous, of the progress and diffusion of physical knowledge. One is, the boldness of modern hypotheses in regard to the highest problems of the Universe and of Man—a boldness sanctioned, it may be, by successes attained, and by the power derived from new agents and methods of research. The other is, the more general and rigid demand for *evidence* on every subject of enquiry, resulting from these methods of research, and not limited to physical science only, but extending to other and very dissimilar questions in which truth is the object sought for. I can affirm a change in the strictness of this demand for *proof* even within my own time. It is much more obvious when comparing the methods and the logic now applied to a disputed question, with those of a century or two centuries ago. This change, familiar as a fact to all who take note of the aspects and bearings of modern enquiry, cannot be too highly appreciated, seeing that its effect must be to discard all spurious knowledge, and at the same time better to define those limits which form an insuperable barrier to human reason.

To pass at once from these generalities to a very different and more special influence on society, viz., that derived from the inordinate multiplication of the London Clubs—institutions absorbing much of the time and talent which might else be given to domestic life, or to life in other forms. The growth of the last forty years as regards the number and palatial magnificence of their buildings, they mark a particular phase of society, and one in which good and evil are doubtfully blended. Ephemeral reading, with frequent interludes of sleep on well-cushioned arm-chairs, and the τί καινόν? question and talk of the day, will probably be admitted by those conversant with Clubs as a fair general picture of their interior life, exclusively of what belongs to the business of the dining-rooms. The latter, except when brought into competition with plainer tables at home, merit more commendation ; contrasted as they are with the grosser conditions of life in the old London taverns and lodging-houses fifty years ago. Refinements in food and furniture may err from excess, but their salutary influence is not to be disregarded. Every man is moulded more or less by his daily surroundings, and the vulgar eye becomes insensibly refined by the fairer forms and colours brought before it.

I must not, however, dilate on this matter of the London Clubs, of which my own knowledge is very partial.

I never have belonged to any other than the Athenæum ;
and though a member of this almost from its origin,
have made much scantier use than most members do of
the various advantages it affords, and never since 1830
have taken any active part in its business.   In that year
I was chosen one of a Committee of thirteen (I am now
the sole survivor of the number), appointed to select, by
unanimity of vote, one hundred out of the many hundred candidates on the books, to be immediately admitted as members.   This *selection* came in priority to
the *election* by the Club at large of a hundred more.
The distinction between the two modes of admission
was keenly appreciated ; and the eager struggle to be
among the *select*, curiously illustrated a frequent form
of human foible.   The business of the Committee,
pledged to unanimity, was laborious, litigious and encumbered with much correspondence; and I was well
pleased when it came to an end.   A voyage to Russia
immediately afterwards showed me *unanimity* obtained
by much more summary and stringent methods of
reaching an object designed.   It will be long before
the Clubs—political, military and literary—of Pall Mall,
find their rivals in the great Nevski Street of St.
Petersburg.

Mr. Croker was the Chairman of the Committee just
mentioned ; and his astute but despotic energy, well
known to all who knew the man, was shown in the way in
which he carried the selection of any candidate for whom
he was interested.   His mere methods might have been
an amusing study to an indifferent observer.   In one

case indeed he failed, though putting out all his powers both of pressure and persuasion. The admission of another person of some public note, was so strongly contested, that I myself received letters from four Cabinet Ministers canvassing me warmly for him. The contest in this case ended in election.

Unless singularity be a merit, I can claim no credit for my feelings and habits as to elections generally. Though comprehending their necessity and value in a free country, I nevertheless have practically abstained from taking part in them, wherever this has been possible. I say it with some shame that, having had the right of voting for Members of Parliament for more than half a century, I have never once exercised this right. It is not likely that I should now ever do so. My personal experience of political elections, curiously enough, has been greater in the United States than in England ; and I am bound to say that that experience (embracing the preparatory stages both of Presidential and municipal elections) has not contributed to reconcile me to them.*

If any method could be discovered for sustaining the life and liberties of a great people, whether England or England's progeny, without having recourse to these periodical popular appeals, I for one should hail the

---

* I speak here of *preparatory stages*, because the final acts of election in the United States are not otherwise defaced than by breaches, more or less frequent, in the integrity of the ballot. The long and passionate party struggles which precede these elections, giving mischievous scope to men who make a traffic of political principles and places, these are the blemishes of a system which has so much that is noble in its origin and design.

discovery. But in the actual state of the world I cannot conjecture any.

To revert, however, to the general question of comparison between this generation and the one preceding it. Though depending on details seemingly within reach of all, yet can this question never be solved by the commonplace phrases current on the subject. It is a difficult one even to those who are able to free themselves from the besetting ambiguities of language, of habits, and of personal relations. The mind unconsciously takes up partial instances in proof—different minds measure proofs differently—and the conclusions attainable are generally too vague to be of value either for speculation or practical use.

To one change within my own lifetime, and this still in progress, I have already slightly adverted. It is, the closer intermingling of the higher and middle classes of Society—the effect in part of the improved education and augmented wealth of the latter; but due also to other causes, such as the altered constitution of the House of Commons; the multiplication of public meetings and societies of every kind and purport; Clubs, Joint Stock Companies, &c., all tending to the fusion of classes before dissociated. Even the modern methods of travelling may be concerned in the result; as well as those changes in ordinary apparel, which among professional men as well as others have abolished many of the distinctions formerly accepted in the world. Whether what Shakespeare in one of his finest passages calls the neglection of degree,' and reproves as such, be for good or evil, I will not here assume to say, though inclining strongly to the latter belief. But the fact is one which we are bound to recognise, and abide the results.*

I may mention in the same cursory way another change manifest to me during my London life, and in truth hardly less obvious in the world at large. This is (using the word here in its simpler sense) the increased *fastness* of living, incident to all classes and occupations of men. Looking especially at home, we find that the augmented speed and hurry of locomotion (and I can affirm that people walk *faster* in the London streets than they did when I first knew these great thoroughfares) is carried into every other department of life ; politics, commerce, literature, science, professional and social existence. The loiterers in life are fewer, and the charm of a tranquil leisure is less appreciated and sought after. The country life of England has also undergone various alteration. Country-houses, if not left vacant for the year, are peopled for a shorter time than heretofore. The relations of landlords to tenants, of masters to servants, of the farmer to his labourers, have all been modified by the new conditions to which

---

* I would fain utter a few words of remonstrance, however, against that assumption of *vulgarities* of dress, now so prevalent among English gentlemen. A mere affectation in many cases, it does not conciliate the classes whose dress is copied, and tends more or less to vulgarise the higher qualities of the wearer. It must be a strong mind which is wholly free from the influences of outward apparel. Though many more potent causes are at work in altering the relations of classes in our time, this may be admitted among the minor influences concerned.

they are submitted. Without going into other details or reasoning on the social effects of these changes, I mention them as facts which must be obvious to all who take any note of the current and course of the human tide flowing beside them.

And I may here allude to another conspicuous change, belonging to the period of my own life, and never more strongly marked than at the present time. I mean, the state of religious thought and action throughout the nation at large. When I first attended to this subject—and I did so somewhat early in life—there was what might be termed a state of religious quietude,—stagnation it would now be called. The established Clergy might be divided broadly into the Arminian and Calvinistic—the former more numerous, the latter more energetic. The English Catholic body was then comparatively small and inert. It had not yet become a proselytizing one. The chief subjects of controversy in our own Church were the doctrines of the Trinity, Original Sin, Atonement and Predestination—disputes which few divines would willingly reopen at the present day.* Some excitement was added to them by the secession about this time of Mr. Lindsay and two or three other Clergymen from the Established Church, in expression of their dissent from the doctrines just named.*

---

* Among these controversial writings I recollect to have been much interested by one under the name of Gregory Blunt, but attributed to Porson, and bearing many marks of his caustic talent. It was an answer to a tract of Granville Sharp, who had undertaken a vindication of Bishop Middleton's argument for the Trinity, from the collocation of the Greek article in certain texts of Scripture.

Still it was a comparative calm, until suddenly disturbed by the Tractarian movement some thirty years ago; the progress and ulterior results of which I have no need to mention here, further than as marking the great change to which I have adverted. These prior controversies have been exchanged—and unhappily with greater excitement — for such as relate to the Real Presence, Baptismal Regeneration, and the several Sacraments ; to the Apostolic succession, Church History, Ritualism, &c. —topics in which the very principles of the Reformation are obviously and deeply concerned. Another subject of controversy, viz., the question as to Scriptural Inspiration, has been revived under the growth of that more subtle sceptical spirit which, whether derived or not from the methods and teachings of physical science, has applied itself to every department of human enquiry, and will continue to do so. Declining, as I must, all speculation as to the causes and future results of the changes just described, I am bound to notice one present good arising out of them, in the increased zeal and activity of the Clergy at large—an effect made known to me professionally as well as by general observation. These qualities would be still more beneficial in their influence were they less alloyed by those sectarian struggles and hatreds which dishonour religion now, as they have done at every preceding period of ecclesiastical history. While simply stating these things as I see them, I do not desire to pursue the subject further.

Passing from these graver topics, I may supplement

what I have before said in comparison of the literary character of the two periods, by taking a single element of society—the 'Wits,' for instance, who held sway as such in the last generation. During the earlier part of my London life, I was in habits of constant intimacy with many men thus designated, though several of them were eminent also for other and higher endowments, Without seeking to lengthen the list, I may mention the names of Canning, Sydney Smith, Jekyll, Lord Alvanley, Lord Dudley, Hookham Frere, Luttrell, Rogers, and Theodore Hook, as well representing the contemporaneous wits of that time with whom I was acquainted. The day of Sheridan had already closed in gloom, and I do not recollect ever to have seen him in society.

But how difficult to define even the word *Wit* itself as the basis of the question ! Graduating downwards from its original and loftier meaning (a transition the steps of which it is amusing to follow), it has come to denote a dozen different qualities and shades of that which the mind receives through its sense of the ridiculous—a faculty as definite as others that we write and read upon in intellectual philosophy, and therefore, as Dr. Johnson has said of it, 'lawfully to be used.' When Cicero— hardly to be called a witty man himself, though in his Epistles sometimes approaching it—talks of and defines the *duplex jocandi genus*, his distinction refers mainly to the moral use of the faculty; without regard to those diversities of humour which are curiously embodied in the social intercourse of mankind, and serve so much to invigorate, if not also to refine, it.

Of the men just named, scarcely two were witty exactly in the same vein. In Jekyll and Hook the talent of the simple punster predominated, but in great perfection of the art; while Bishop Blomfield and Baron Alderson, whom I have often seen in friendly conflict, enriched this art by the high classical accomplishments they brought to it. The wit of Lord Dudley, Lord Alvanley, and Rogers, was poignant personal sarcasm;—in Luttrell it was perpetual fun, of lighter and more various kind, and whimsically expressed in his features as well as his words. *Natio comœda est* was the maxim of his mind and denoted the wide field of his humour. The wit of Mr. Canning was of rarer and more refined workmanship, and drew larger ornament from classical sources. The 'Anti-Jacobin' shows Mr. Canning's power in its youthful exuberance. When I knew him it had been sobered, perhaps saddened, by the political contrarieties and other incidents of more advanced life, but had lost none of its refinement of irony. Less obvious than the common wit of the world, it excited thought and refined it—one of the highest characteristics of this faculty.

The vein of humour in Hookham Frere, like that of his and my friend William Rose, was strongly tinged with the style of the Italian romantic poetry of the fifteenth century, that of Ariosto, Boiardo, Casti, &c. His strange poem of 'Whistlecraft,' coloured in this serio-comic fashion, put at defiance all common comprehension, and was indeed very little known or read. He counted upon the saying of Lord Shaftesbury, 'that it is a dull sort of wit which amuses all alike,' and in this spirit rather enjoyed, I think, the failure of his poem. His translations from Simonides, almost in the boyhood of life, show how early his powers as a poet were evoked. But Frere's chief revelry when I knew him was in Aristophanes ; and his translations of that great comic writer, though fragmentary, mark the strong hold he had got of the spirit as well as text of his author. When in London, he used frequently to send me proof-slips of these several translations, fresh from the press. His peculiar vein of humour did not suggest any fitness for a diplomatist ; but his intimate connection with Mr. Canning twice brought him forward in this capacity. His second appointment on a mission to Spain, at an early and critical period of the great Peninsular War was somewhat severely commented upon at the time. He gained no glory from his diplomacy, but was careless about it.*

His life afterwards, whether in England or in Malta where he died, became an indolent intellectuality, with a sort of sarcastic indifference to fame and to the bustling world around him. In conversation always animated and pleasant, he yet found his chief happiness in the quiet of old books and whimsical reveries, the '*inertes horæ*' of the poet. His strange absences of mind were the subject of some amusing anecdotes

* A saying attributed to Mr. Frere, that he loved Spain 'as a country in which God had so much land in his own holding' has the true tone of his humour about it. He was created 'Marquis of Union' by the Supreme Junta before his departure; but irrespectively of other reasons, no man was so little likely to bring this title into use.

among the few with whom he continued in habits of
intercourse. He knew and humorously vindicated his
own indolence, in its contrast with the angry and
agitated lives of many of his political friends. Some
good might be gained to the busy life of our own
days by the larger admixture in it of this more
tranquil element of character. The faculty of being
happy when alone, though derived chiefly from natural
temperament, is susceptible of more cultivation than it
receives, and will well repay whatever culture can be
given to it. But the torrent of the world, especially at
this time, is such and so strong that few can escape
being drawn into its vortex.

A word must be given to James Smith, the author of
the 'Rejected Addresses,' as one among the wits of the
time of which I am speaking. His jovial temperament,
expressed in face and figure, was always ready to
expend itself in society, for his own enjoyment as well
as that of others. The profusion with which he poured
forth his humorous ballads one after another, in a rich
and resonant voice, came in curious contrast to the
fastidiousness of Moore, who scrutinised his audience
carefully before he could be persuaded to sing. The
'Rejected Addresses' have survived longer than most
parodies, and justifiably so; for there is a fine poetical
element in this work, underlying the excellence of the
parodies themselves and enriching them.

If I were seeking to describe the *witty women* of this
period, I should not hesitate to place Lady Morley
at the head of them. To a keen sense of the ludicrous

in personal character and social life, she added the adornment of much classical reading, highly cultivated taste, and great felicity of expression. Yet, though thus richly provided, her wit was never 'willing to wound,' even when most tempted by the oddities or follies of which she had so quick an apprehension. Many are yet remaining to confirm what I here say of Lady Morley. Her printed pieces, though short and scattered, attest the rare merits of her humour. The 'Petition of the Hens of Great Britain to the House of Commons against the Importation of French Eggs' is an excellent specimen of them. So are her letters to Sydney Smith, which reciprocate fully the various wit redundant in his part of the correspondence. The excellence of Lady Morley's character in private life, which I had much opportunity of seeing, was in no wise lessened by those other accomplishments which gave to her so great a charm in society.

I cannot quit this allusion to the witty women of this time without again mentioning the three daughters of Lord North, to whom their talent of playful, inoffensive humour came as a happy family inheritance.* The same talent, aided by many other lovable qualities, made the house of Catherine Fanshawe in Berkeley Square one of the familiar resorts of the literary men of the day. These quiet coteries, blending literature with general society, dispensing with cards of invitation and other formalities, and (what is essential to their well-being), having a lady for the hostess—are fewer, I think, and

* Lady Glenborvie, Lady Sheffield, and Lady Charlotte Lindsay.

less frequented than they used to be, and more hampered by the technicalities of London life. The probable explanation is to be found in that miscellaneous crowding of all society, to which I have before alluded.

If mentioning the name of Sydney Smith apart from those already noted, it is because I think the power and diversity of his wit—taking the term in its largest sense—greater than that of any man I have ever known. I might seek from my intimate knowledge of him to point out its more signal characteristics, some perhaps which have escaped general notice ; but all that can be conveyed by writing has been already well and faithfully given by one dear to him and to myself ; and no new description could come nearer to that reality, which every year there are fewer to recollect. The 'Wit and Wisdom of Sydney Smith' is the title of a book first published on the other side of the Atlantic, where his writings are as thoroughly appreciated as in England. It pithily expresses what peculiarly belongs to them. For underneath the almost riotous exuberance of his humour, joyous to himself as to all around him, there ever lay a foundation of strong masculine sense, as well as of wholesome satire upon the foibles or wrongdoings of the world. Intellect is essential to true wit, as the name implies ; and no one, not even Rabelais or Swift, ever brought them into closer combination. It is a conjunction peculiar to man. The dog and the monkey have a keen sense of *fun* ; but the refinements of wit are as purely characteristic of man as are the highest attainments of learning or science.

There is one peculiarity about Sydney Smith as a writer (having some kindred indeed with wit), which I think has not been enough noticed. I mean the *unexpectedness* of his style, and the entire carelessness as to method and ornament if his object is well reached. He rarely deals either with preface or peroration, but grasps at once the matter in hand, and stops when he has no more to say. Swift somewhere speaks of ' the Ghost of Wit delighting to walk after the death of the body.' Sydney Smith's writings are never haunted by this spirit. His wit comes unsought for, serves its purpose, and he passes at once again into serious argument—serious, but always short and pithy in style. Those who love Dryden—and they ought to be legion—will recognise the charm belonging to the bold and unexpected phrases of his poetry. Sydney Smith's prose has the same charm. His phrases are never pedantic or pirated, but always fresh from the mint of his own genius. He never looked over again what he had once written, and, as I know, could hardly ever be persuaded to correct the errors of a proof-sheet. He revelled in his own manner of handling a subject, and was comparatively careless of its effect on others.

One of his warmest admirers was the late President Lincoln, who more than once has quoted to me passages from his writings which I had forgotten. Lincoln was himself a man of much quaint humour, curiously expressed in tales of Kentucky and Illinois life, told in their broadest form of American speech. These he brought into connection with events seeming to require a graver illustration, yet which could not really have been better illustrated. Of the six Presidents of the United States whom I have known, including Andrew Johnson, he seemed to me the only one gifted with this faculty. I recollect sitting with him and Mr. Seward over a log-fire in the White House (the Federal forts and General Lee's dismantled villa seen from the windows across the Potomac), a few hours only after intelligence had been received of the first disastrous battle of Chattanooga. The conversation at first centred on this event; but the cheerful temperament of these two remarkable men gradually transferred it to other topics; and the President amused himself and us by some of those racy anecdotes which so often convey more of practical truth than any dry reasoning can afford—now and then stopping for a moment to put a fresh log on the fire. The possession of this simple and genial humour, not alloyed by any personal asperities, helped greatly that popularity, which was mainly due to the honesty and consistency of the man, in times of unforeseen and perilous trial to his country. The constant and cordial support which he and my friend Mr. Seward, in their respective positions, gave to each other during this long and arduous struggle, greatly contributed, as I believe, to its successful termination. The latter, though severely wounded by the weapon of the assassin, maintained his vigour of purpose and action to the end.*

---

* Speaking thus much of President Lincoln, I may add that I possess the map of the seat of war in Virginia which he himself habitually used

I find, however, that I am unawares straying too far from the course of my narrative ; and, though unwillingly, must bring it back to my own more immediate concerns. Of events indeed, excluding as I do all family history, I have little more to relate in a life which has been singularly exempt from worldly accidents or anxieties. The term *sensational* has crept or rather forced itself into modern use. My life has yielded little to which this word can rightly be applied. What I may yet find to say will have relation chiefly to those private occupations and habits, often indeed colouring life more deeply and lastingly than the rarer events which seem for a time to illumine or darken it.

for reference. He gave it to me on my return home from the headquarters of the Army of the Potomac, writing his name and mine on the margin of the map. His affectionate farewell to me when I left Washington I cannot easily forget. Three years afterwards I stood on the very spot of his assassination. The theatre in which it occurred was then in progress of conversion into a Pathological Museum ; recording by the specimens on its shelves the camp-diseases of the war just come to an end, and the strange wounds inflicted by new and more fatal instruments of warfare. While I was examining these, a poor soldier came in, his arm amputated above the elbow-joint, praying to be allowed to look for a moment at his ' *old elbow*,' which had already taken its place among the other specimens in the Museum. The affectionate recognition of his old joint, and the curious terms of endearment applied to it, rendered this really a touching incident.

CHAPTER XI.

I HAVE hitherto spoken of my connection with the persons and society of a generation passing away, or indeed almost gone by. While refraining, for what I think just reasons, from any similar notices of individuals now living, I may venture to say of myself, that I have preserved and enjoyed the same relations of social intercourse with the present generation as with the past—altered indeed as to persons, and in certain respects as to the fashions of life, but alike in general character, and with no change to myself that I could feel as an abrupt disseverment of former ties. Preserving, as I have happily been able to do, the same habits and occupations, I have passed quietly from one period to another with little actual consciousness of change, save at those times when the memory has accidentally been led to some sudden and wider retrospect of the life already gone by. Of harsh lines of contrast there have been none. The preservation of health has doubtless contributed much to this result : but I willingly claim something also as due to the maintenance of those pursuits, not merely professional in kind, which have kept me in association with men eminent in the literature and science of the day, and with their writings and discoveries. It is a true though very trite remark, that such persevering occupation is the best solace to the tedium and other ills of advancing life. The mind often needs to be rescued from itself, and nothing can do this so easily or so well.

At the risk of appearing egotistical, I may indulge myself here in a few details, pleasant as memories, and useful perhaps prospectively to some of my many grandchildren and others now beginning life. I will not put them among the *verba otiosorum senum ad imperitos juvenes*, as I am still somewhat short of the *otiosus senex* myself—but near enough to it to warrant a few notices and suggestions derived from the experience of an active life. I begin, however, by a suggestion applying rather to the old than to the young, and little more indeed than an enforcement of what I have just said.

There is a certain acquiescence in, and adaptation to, the several stages of advancing years, which every wise man will recognise as the fitting sequel to what has gone before. The καλῶς σχολάζειν is a happy phrase in its application to any age, but especially to that of waning life. The changes however so required, if now and then adopted too late, are often in my belief made prematurely—either from distrust and disuse of the natural powers still left, or from the tyranny of habits successively encroaching upon them. The want of occupation is, according to my experience professional as well as social a very frequent cause of premature decay. Cicero said this long ago, but his sonorous phrases somewhat obscure the practical part of the maxim. Retirement from business and quietude of life are happy provisions, taken at the right time and in the right degree. But they may be adopted too soon, and too largely indulged in ; and the vitality both of mind and body be unduly impaired by the very means employed to preserve it. Easy arm-chairs and other appliances of luxurious comfort are an invitation to indolence, and to the disuse of faculties which need employment for their preservation. I have sometimes succeeded in rescuing patients from this premature decrepitude, where the habits it involves have not taken too deep root. The encroachment of such habits needs to be sedulously watched, for they always come on insidiously, and grow both on body and mind by indulgence. *Peu de gens savent être vieux* is an expression of much truth, though coming from a cynical quarter. A higher French authority, speaking of *cet inexorable ennui qui fait le fond de la vie humaine*, well adds that occupation alone can preserve us from it. The weariness of life is, in truth, one of its greatest pains ; from which even highly gifted men have sometimes sought relief by bringing life itself to an end. The physician sees much of all these things, but there is yet more unseen.

My own convictions on this subject have led me to keep up sedulously, even to the present time (and I am writing when more than eighty) all the occupations and habits which were most congenial to me when young, or have subsequently become so. As regards the *bodily part* of these habits, a good constitution not impaired by excesses, together with a certain amount of *determination* on the subject, have preserved to me more of activity than is common at my age ; of which the ability, still continued, of undertaking long and somewhat arduous journeys is sufficient evidence.* But with all this I do not forget Lord Bacon's pithy expression, 'a healthy old man is a tower undermined,' and shall strive to take early warning of changes as they successively occur. Some predetermination is necessary for this, and a fair allowance for the collateral incidents of life. The *intellecta senectus* is a happy phrase of Juvenal in its bearing on the whole condition of old age.

With respect to intellectual habits, I have already spoken of the resolution formed on entering professional life, to maintain, as far as could be done, the various pursuits which then most interested me. Having early learnt, from some striking examples, how hard it is to fulfil this purpose under the strain of a busy medical career, I sought to do so partly, as before mentioned, by putting a certain limit to this professional absorption,— partly by methodising somewhat minutely, but in no way harshly, my habits as to these other occupations. One or two instances will show the sort of rule I

---

* Trifling instances are often the best in illustration. A frequent source of amusement to myself is my *incapacity* for walking slowly ; and the sort of compulsion I even now feel to pass those immediately before me in the street, and to take the diagonal instead of the two sides of a square, whenever this is the alternative. I mentioned the latter circumstance to my excellent friend Mr. Richmond, when he was finishing a crayon-portrait of me. 'You ought,' he said, 'to have told me this before.' When I cease to take the diagonal (often a dirty one) instead of the side pavements, I shall consider that I have gone a step downwards in the path of life.

adopted long ago, and have beneficially persevered in even to the present time.

My classical education, in the common use of the phrase, was a very imperfect one, for I do not believe I ever made a tolerable set of Latin verses. But it imbued me with sufficient love of the great writers of Greece and Rome to carry me forward into private study of them; and this study, ripened by time and my travels in classical lands, has become a source of ever-increasing enjoyment. My recollections furnish me with a little history of the stages of appreciation at successive periods of life, attesting its increase even to the moment at which I am now writing. I have just finished my third reading of the 'Odyssey' under the feeling of augmented pleasure, and have passed on to the very dissimilar reading of the 'Wasps' of Aristophanes ; with less pleasure indeed, but still with much amusement in seeking to unravel the whimsical web of Athenian social life, at once so unlike and so like that of our own day.

Many, perhaps all, who have held fast to these studies must have noted in themselves the same result of increasing pleasure in their pursuit. But no long gap must be allowed, or the faculty of enjoyment is lost, and rarely regained. It is an old but true remark, that the greatest works, whether of art or literature, do not at once disclose their full perfection to the eye or understanding. They are mines of discovery, the richer the deeper they are worked. Equally is it true that a certain maturity of age and knowledge is necessary to reach and thoroughly compass these deeper workings. A youth fresh from school or college may have read the ' Iliad ' and the ' Prometheus,' and yet know little of Homer or Æschylus. He may have select passages from Lucretius and half of Horace in his memory, and yet be unable to comprehend the sublimity of the former, or the *curiosa felicitas* of the latter. This remark stands good for the great classics of all ages— for Dante, Shakespeare, and Milton—but I adduce it here only as regards my own experience on the subject.

At the time when my medical practice most pressed on other occupations, I maintained these studies by the methods alluded to, which I may here briefly explain. They are simple indeed in kind, and might easily have been lost amidst the business and entanglements of life ; but a steady perseverance has given to them the force of habit—that strongest of all forces. I allotted three days each week to Greek and Latin reading, under the resolution never to let the day pass wholly without it, even though but ten minutes could be kept free from other business. Every day, even the busiest, will yield its ten minutes over and over again, if they are well looked after and taken up at the time ; and such sudden change of employment is made easy by habit, and often indeed refreshing to the mind.* Carrying Latin and Greek

* I have much aided myself in using these *fractions* of time by the practice, now of forty years' standing, of transcribing into a volume, with a certain classification of subjects, all the finest passages of Greek and Latin poetry and prose which have come under my own reading. This practice I have kept up to the present moment, having added even to-day some lines from the *Andromache* of Euripides to what are probably a couple of thousand passages from different authors, already in this volume. To these I ever come with pleasure, due not solely to their intrinsic value, but also

books with me in my carriage, till my eyes refused the
latter, I have found no difficulty in passing at once from
the sorrows of Iphigenia or Dido to the ailments and
plaints of a sick-room in Grosvenor Square; and even a
genial connection in coming fresh from Horace, Catullus,
or Lucretius, to the men of wit or learning with whom as
patients I have been so often associated. The practice
of a West-end physician in London abounds, in truth,
in cases which give little occasion for thought or solici-
tude, and are best relieved by a frequent half-hour of
genial conversation; while in those more serious, the
patient does not suffer by the physician bringing to his
bedside a mind disengaged from the other maladies that
have just been under his eye, or pressed anxiously on
his consideration. Without presuming, then, to say how
it may be with other physicians—for no two minds are
exactly alike in this, or anything else—I venture to
speak of the diversion of thought so obtained as having
been salutary to myself, and in no way injurious, as I
believe, to my patients.

This habit of methodised reading has carried me
through a larger range of ancient writers than perhaps

to my long familiarity with them as thus transcribed by myself. To give a
readable value to such a volume, the extracts must be short, and the writing,
especially of the Greek passages, clear and good. To the latter essential
point I have sedulously attended. I take up this volume whenever prevented from more consecutive reading, sure when I open it to find abundant
enjoyment. Similar enjoyment I have had from another manuscript
volume, ever at hand, containing numerous select passages from old
English prose writers, derived chiefly from my own reading. These
passages, in their antiquated style and modes of thought, afford a pleasure
which Pope has somewhat whimsically compared to that of travelling over
an old Roman way.

is usual among amateur students of the classics—including, for instance, the later Latin poets and historians, and some of the Byzantine writers of still later
date. The very absence of anything like nice or critical
scholarship has enabled me to wander cursorily over
these wider but more barren fields, without impairing
my enjoyment of the higher works of ancient genius. It
is true, as Dr. Johnson says, that 'snatches of reading do
not make a Bentley or a Clarke;' but to those, like
myself, not scholars by profession, or aiming at this
high grade of learning, these little excursions out of the
common course fill up the gaps of other studies, and
illustrate agreeably the various phases of human
life at successive periods. It is a trifling case in point,
but I may mention that I have lately been pleasantly
occupied with the two poems on the Dog—the Cyne-
getica of Gratius and Nemesianus — my love for the
animal lending a lively interest to these ancient records
of his habits and virtues. The character of the dog
has undergone less change than that of the human
master to whom he is so strangely attached.

At this time, when the question is agitated as to the
methods of classical education in England, I would
venture the remark, that our usage assigns too narrow a
scope to the study of ancient authors, whether at College or afterwards. I have known, for instance, men of
high reputed scholarship who had never looked into the
physical writings of Aristotle, marvellous productions for
any age—nor into what remains of the great Astronomical Poem of Aratus, quoted by St. Paul, and trans-

lated by Cicero in his youth—nor into the orations of
Isæus, the master of Demosthenes and ' the great pro-
perty-lawyer of antiquity ;' — and who were wholly
unread in the first and tenth chapters of Quintilian—the
first an excellent treatise on education, having much in
common with Locke ; the other one of the finest pieces
of literary criticism extant.   These instances are slight
in themselves, but they will serve to show what I mean
under much wider application.   The strict demand for
the niceties of versification at our public schools has
doubtless contributed to this result ; repelling many in
the outset ; and limiting the reading of others to the
authors received as models of the different styles.*

On the days alternate to those given to Greek and
Latin reading, I have pursued a similar plan as to German and Italian, but with less close adherence to rule.
During my early travels on the Continent, I committed
to memory a large amount of Italian, and a good deal
of German poetry ; and very much of this I still retain
as a pleasurable possession of later life.   Such especially
I have always found it when travelling alone, or in places
where some distraction of thought or feeling was required.
The frequent or indeed habitual recourse at such times
to this early stock of poetry, has kept it well together in

---

* Physical science is not often associated with classical reading.   Yet
the wonderful poem of Lucretius ought, in one form or other, to be more
frequently in the hands of all who are now working at the development of
the Atomic and Molecular theory.   Scarcely a step made in advance in
this research, which has not in some sort been shadowed forth by this great
poet ; either on his own inspiration, or that of the Greek philosopher to
whom he pays such splendid homage.

my memory, while later acquisitions of the same kind have wholly passed away. Even for the more common-place object of courting sleep, when it is reluctant to come, these poetical recollections have served me better than any of the ordinary devices for that purpose. I have a large provision of Dante always at hand for such use; but I find it easier and more luxurious to steal into slumber through a sonnet of Petrarch, or the stanzas of Ariosto and Tasso. The sonnet is perhaps the most effective soporific, in whatever language it be written.

On the principle already referred to, of maintaining my earlier pursuits, as well as from a deep interest in the physical sciences, now pressing so rapidly onward, I have devoted a certain time each day to some one or other of these; well knowing that the continuity of pursuit here, once thoroughly broken, can rarely be recovered. As in the case of classical reading, a very short time regularly applied suffices to fulfil the purpose. I have practically felt the advantage of this rule; which, though incompetent to deal with the copious details, ever augmenting, of each science, has yet enabled me to keep pace with all the greater discoveries of the day, and especially with those researches tending to give connection and unity to the different sciences—the method by which nearest approach is made to the great mysteries of the universe. To those whose professional objects have kept them out of the direct path of experimental research, this correlation of the physical sciences becomes itself an ample field for thought and enquiry. It is a science in itself.

For the sake of my readers, whatever their age, I would fain put in a few words more, regarding the value of these disposable fractions of time of which I have spoken, in the economy of life. Where the habitual occupation is grave and laborious, they may sometimes be accepted as a 'wise idleness'—a void left for tranquil thought or reverie, and recovery of exhausted power. But in far the majority of cases these lesser portions of time—the 'moments which make the year'—are idly frittered away, and practically lost to life. '*Le temps c'est la vie*' is a terse expression of a great truth ; and the accumulative value of its fractional parts has never been more happily illustrated than by the wit of Sydney Smith—here as elsewhere based on practical wisdom.* Quintilian, ever full of such wisdom, has strikingly expressed the sort of living suicide men commit upon themselves by this neglect of time, '*Breve nobis tempus nos facimus.*' Life requires to be analysed in its several parts to gain a fitting knowledge of their relative value ; and such analysis may be usefully repeated at intervals as life goes on.

Without pretending to have made adequate use of my own stray leisure, I have always sought to regard it as a beneficial property in hand, and have found great good

---

* Addressing a young lady, he says, ' Do you ever reflect how you pass your life ? If you live to seventy-two, which I hope you may, your life is passed in the following manner : An hour a day is three years. This makes twenty-seven years sleeping ; nine years dressing ; nine years at table ; six years playing with children ; nine years walking, drawing, and visiting ; six years shopping, and three years quarrelling.' I have heard him similarly estimate for himself the portion of life he had spent in shaving, always a long occupation with him.

from so doing. In this I have been somewhat aided by what I can only recommend under much qualification— viz., the desultory character of my reading. Apart from those subjects which I have noticed as more or less methodised into daily occupation, I have generally kept three or four books simultaneously in hand, without any regard to congruity of topics; or rather indeed expressly seeking for diversity in this respect. Even Novels—that exuberant growth of late years, almost setting a mark on the time in which we live—have fairly come in among graver books; and by not craving for the newest, I have generally in the end got the best. My friend Lord Dudley used to say, that he spared himself a great deal both of reading and talking by patiently waiting till the fashionable book of the day had '*blown over*'—a rule which might beneficially apply to many cases in life besides that of ephemeral reading. Every topic of public talk is now fast hurried away in the torrent of passing events.

As regards novels, I could not cross-examine my children in the family history of Sir Charles Grandison and Harriet Byron, as Lord Macaulay sometimes did, and was well able to do in the most minute details of dress and demeanour. But I am sufficiently versed in them to be able to admire the amount of human talent given to these delineations of human life—to the de- picturing of men and women through fictions addressed chiefly to the sensational part of our nature. Those of highest merit may well take rank with the best poetry of the age, and there are many which well deserve this relative position. Of the general moral effects of this literature—for good or for ill—I do not assume to judge, or at least need not speak here. It unquestionably has usurped largely upon other and more profitable reading; and includes much which had better not be read at all.

With resources so far various, I have never found difficulty in filling up the smaller fractions of time, thus valuable in their totality, with some subject that suited the inclinations or aptitudes of the moment. I must repeat that this fashion of reading cannot be recommended without reserve, especially where there is any serious matter in hand. But while mentioning it only as one that has served well and agreeably to myself, I may add that the power of passing promptly from one subject to another, is a faculty not to be despised, or even neglected, as a point in mental education. It is one form of that *command* of the mind over its own acts and associations, which tends to produce the highest as well as most useful forms of intellectual life. The strongest minds may be not only wearied but weakened by too intent direction to one subject; and change in such cases is wisdom and not fickleness. *Levat lassitudinem laboris mutatio* is the phrase of one of the wisest of Roman physicians. In practice I have often had occasion to found my advice on this precept—in some cases even where a wranglership at Cambridge was endangered by the counsel given.

I have never been a book-collector, as regards either the number, or the quality and rarity of the volumes I possess. My library, in truth, hardly deserves to be called such. Nearly half of it, and the only valuable part, consists of works given to me by their authors or others ; and these I leave collectively to my eldest Son. It is pleasant to me to count among the books which I owe to their authors, the works of Walter Scott, Macaulay, Hallam, Milman, Wordsworth, the Duc d'Aumale, Lord Stanhope, Whewell, Guizot, Miss Edgeworth, Henry Taylor, Joanna Baillie, Everett, Prescott, &c. ; Southey made me one of the private recipients of his anonymous work *The Doctor* ; curious as a miscellany of various learning, but wanting the felicitous humour of Rabelais and Sterne. I possess three translations of the ' Iliad '— those of Lord Derby, Sir John Herschel, and Mr. Sotheby —each the gift of the translator. Lord Derby's volumes need no commendation from me. Sir J. Herschel has done all that genius could do to rescue English hexameter verse from the reproach of Roger Ascham, that ' it doth rather trot and hobble than run smoothly in our tongue.' It may well be kept in mind in this case that it was the same genius which successfully accosted so many of the most profound problems in physical science. I have already mentioned Sir J. Herschel as one of the very few whom I have known, blending high literary attainments and a strong poetic feeling with these sterner pursuits.*

---

* A few months only have elapsed since this admirable man was lost to us—lost to science, it may well be said, for no one ever brought to physical inquiry in all its branches more knowledge and genius, conjoined with an integrity and candour which are never found save in those who love truth

The remainder of my library, though including various medical literature, would furnish but a few hours' work to the book-sales through which so many great libraries, the collection of years, are suddenly scattered again over the world, to provide the materials for fresh aggregation. My notions indeed as to these large libraries are somewhat heretical. I believe their chief value to consist in the occupation and pleasure afforded by the act of collection; and that very few persons do really read or use the books—other than those of reference—which have gained and hold a place on their book-shelves. The mere fact of being closely at hand deprives them practically of their value. If this be so (and I think it will be found true by those who care, or know how, to examine their own habits), the conclusion is forced upon us that, in a London house at least, books are often the fraudulent occupants of space that might better be left void for air. A family inheritance of folios and quartos, whether in town or country, is generally a very profitless possession. They continue inert and dusty fixtures from one generation to other—a melancholy mockery of the literary toils for which their authors had presaged a happier fate.

I might quote Seneca (a writer whose wisdom is too often hidden by the conceits of his style) as an explicit

---

for truth's sake. I visited him at Collingwood three times in the year preceding his death. The bodily changes going on were too visible. The mind retained its clearness almost to the last; enfeebled indeed as to continuous exertion, but this only by the feebleness of the body. His interment in Westminster Abbey was called for by the unanimous voice of all his most eminent scientific contemporaries.

authority for my heresy on this subject.* He wrote, moreover, when books, as represented by manuscripts, were infinitely less numerous than in our prolific age. The book-shop of the Sosii, near the Temple of Janus, would feebly compare with the literary store of the Longmans near St. Paul's. The *libelli* issuing from the Argiletum Street in Rome were scanty precursors of the volumes from which Albemarle Street derives its reputation. As regards the great public libraries, which count their books by hundreds of thousands, I may say that I never enter one of these huge receptacles without the question pressing on my mind, ' What is it all about ? '—a question short in itself, but admitting of being expanded into a large and curious commentary on the writings of man in every age of the world.

Acting on these impressions, I have given more care to thin my library, such as it is, than to augment it. Each year I devote part of some one day to this special object of *weeding* my books, often summoning fire to my aid in the work. I by no means pretend to put this forward as an example to others. There are some men who gain such *mastery* over their libraries for practical purposes, that it would be a crime to curtail their collections. Such pre-eminently was Lord

---

* *Distringit librorum multitudo. Itaque quum legere non possis quantum habueris, satis est habere quantum legas.*

I have not been successful in converting others to my opinion on this matter. I made indeed a partial convert of Hallam; whom I persuaded to thin his library, by disposal of books which were crowding his house even to unwholesomeness.

Macaulay, of whom one might say what Dryden did of Ben Jonson, 'He invaded authors like a monarch.' Surrounded by his many thousand volumes, he could summon any one to his hands at the moment; and, by a felicity of memory which might well be called instinct, could put his finger almost instantly on the passage sought for. How he used this and his other faculties his works sufficiently tell. No writer had ever his intellectual materials more thoroughly in hand. When his memory failed as to facts it told him at once where to look for them.

A further exception must be made for another friend, Mr. Thomas Grenville, whose library, preserved in all its integrity, is now among the valuable treasures of the British Museum. Mr. Grenville was the latest link with the statesmen of George III.'s reign. The intricate web of family and party connections involved him in some difficulties of position in his earlier career; and later in life the Reform Bill produced some painful disseverments of old friendship, of which I was cognisant. But under none of these circumstances was Mr. Grenville's personal integrity impugned. In his figure and demeanour, as well as in intellect and learning, he was an admirable representative of the high-bred Englishman of any time. His life between eighty and ninety formed a nobler treatise on Old Age than that which Cicero has bequeathed to us.

Had I been a collector of letters, the various correspondence of my long life would itself have given large material for this object. Embracing such habitual correspondents as Hallam, Mackintosh, Macaulay, Jeffrey, Lord Aberdeen, Lady Holland, Whewell, Herschel, Guizot, Everett, &c., with others of more recent date, my collection might have stood fairly in comparison with many of those which the world shows itself eager to accept. But here again, as with regard to books, that which phrenologists might term my 'organ of destructiveness' came into action, and I retain very few indeed of the total number of my letters, and these chiefly to meet the many requests made to me for autographs.* Sydney Smith, who habitually destroyed all he received, vindicated this on the score of conscience towards others. I cannot plead this motive ; nor indeed any more explicit excuse than the belief that a sufficient number will always be left in the world, to meet, even to satiety, any legitimate interest derived from them. Yet I may confess that I now and then feel regret and self-reproach as to this matter, when the memory comes before me of the persons whose letters have been thus destroyed. Those of Lord Aberdeen and Hallam more especially, occurring in close series for many years, and dealing with all public topics of the day, ought to have had another fate.

Though my annual autumnal journeys, after settling

---

* The passion of collecting autographs is not less developed on the other side the Atlantic. The morning after my arrival at Mr. Seward's house in Washington, some years ago, I found eight or ten volumes of such collections lying on my table, with requests that I would write something in each. We are bequeathing to posterity an enormous legacy of autographs and photographs, with little discrimination as to their actual or relative value. Happily, time can obliterate as well as create.

in London, were too rapid, and too vague in their direction, for any actual research, they have greatly aided me in maintaining whatever knowledge of science I had before acquired; and have brought me, as my narrative shows, into connection with many eminent scientific men in different countries. I might refer to Astronomy as an instance of the advantage thus gained—a science in which, though with only casual opportunities for indulging my predilections, I have ever felt especial interest. Some of these opportunities indeed, arising out of my visits to Observatories both in Europe and America, have been remarkable enough to warrant a more particular mention of them.

That which most strongly clings to my memory is an evening I passed with Encke and Galle in the Observatory at Berlin, some ten or twelve days after the discovery of the planet Neptune on this very spot ; and when every night's observations of its motions had still an especial value in denoting the elements of its orbit. I had casually heard of the discovery at Bremen, and lost no time in hurrying on to Berlin. The night in question was one of floating clouds, gradually growing into cumuli ; and hour after hour passed away without sight of the planet which had just come to our knowledge by so wonderful a method of predictive research. Frustrated in this main point, it was some compensation to stay and converse with Encke in his own Observatory, one signalised by so many discoveries—the stillness and darkness of the place broken only by the solemn ticking of the astronomical clock, which, as the unfailing interpreter of the celestial times and motions, has a sort of living existence to the astronomer. Among other things discussed while thus sitting together in a sort of tremulous impatience, was the name to be given to the new planet. Encke told me he had thought of Vulcan; but deemed it right to remit the choice to Leverrier, then supposed the sole indicator of the planet and its place in the heavens—adding that he expected Leverrier's answer by the first post. Not an hour had elapsed before a knock at the door of the Observatory announced the letter expected. Encke read it aloud; and, coming to the passage where Leverrier proposed the name of Neptune, exclaimed, '*So lass den Namen Neptun sein.*' It was a midnight scene not easily to be forgotten. A royal baptism, with its long array of titles, would ill compare with this simple naming of the remote and solitary planet thus wonderfully discovered. There is no place, indeed, where the grandeur and wild ambitions of the world are so thoroughly rebuked, and dwarfed into littleness, as in the Astronomical Observatory.*

I may mention here, that in an article in the 'Quarterly Review' (January 1847) I sought to do justice to the claims of Mr. Adams, in regard to the discovery of

---

* As a practical illustration of this remark, I would add that my own knowledge of Astronomers—those who have worked themselves with the telescope—has shown them to be generally men of tranquil temperament, and less disturbed than others by worldly affairs, or by the quarrels incident even to scientific research. I may mention as instances occurring to me at the moment, the two Herschels, Encke, Bessel, Piazzi and Bond. Other examples might readily be supplied.

the planet Neptune—a point of real interest not solely as relates to this event in the history of science, wonderful though it be, but as affording an index to the principle through which conflicting claims to discovery should be brought to judgment. The case here, indeed, was singularly complex in all its circumstances ; and the only just verdict must be one of *duality* and *equality* of right. So it will stand in the great volume of Astronomical history, that loftiest record of human attainment.

I was at Florence, and in the Observatory of Donati himself, on the very day when the splendid Comet of 1858, named after him, made its nearest approach to the earth. By another coincidence, I dined that evening with my friend Mrs. Somerville—probably the only woman in Europe capable of calculating the orbit of a comet from the elements given by observation. While other ladies at Florence, as I had occasion to know, were purchasing tickets in the State Lottery on some whimsical fancy of numbers connected with the aspects and periods of the Comet, Mrs. Somerville was contemplating it with the eye and knowledge of a philosopher. We looked at this wonderful object together the last evening I passed at Florence. I have never seen Mrs. Somerville since.

My frequent visits to the United States have given me large access to the Observatories there, especially to those of Cambridge, Cincinnati, and Albany. The great Achromatic telescope at Cambridge (the glass of which, 15 inches diameter, I had before seen at

Munich when just completed) became familiar to me when it passed into the use of that admirable observer, Professor Bond, with whom I had frequent communication almost to the end of his life. One of my visits to his Observatory (September 30, 1850) was marked by a fortunate incident. At this time Saturn was in a position singularly favourable for the view of its Rings; and, in fact, the third Ring of the planet was discovered but a few days later, almost simultaneously here and in England—a discovery following after a very short interval that of its eighth Satellite. Mr. Everett and several of the Cambridge Professors were with me in the Observatory that evening, gazing on this grand telescopic object, when we were startled by a sudden burst and blaze of light, illuminating for a moment every corner of the building. Looking out into the night, we saw the still brilliant light of an exploded Meteor, so near to Saturn as to come almost within the same field of telescopic vision— the train stretching over 8° or 10° in length, with a breadth seemingly of little less than a degree—being gradually elongated from a nucleus, and assuming a spiral form or *whorl* at one extremity of this elongation, not unlike some of Lord Rosse's spiral nebulæ—at one time taking on a curious cometary aspect, very much resembling Halley's comet as seen by Sir J. Herschel at the Cape of Good Hope. These singular luminous phenomena were distinctly visible for more than an hour (an unwonted duration of meteoric light), during which time I continued in close observation of them.

A very interesting report on this extraordinary Meteor was made by Professor Bond to the British Association at their Glasgow Meeting in 1855. From connected observations in other parts of Massachusetts, he calculated its height above the earth at the time of its sudden appearance to be about fifty miles. Its rotary motion, on a point answering to the centre of the explosion, was nearly 90° in less than half an hour. From the phenomena of the explosion, there may be some reason to conjecture the fall of an Aerolite at the time; but if so, this fell, as doubtless innumerable aerolites do fall on land and sea, without knowledge or record of them by man.

Alluding to Aerolites, let me add that, having *steamed* through the Dardanelles three several times, I have each time felt a certain compunction in passing unexplored the spot near Lamsaki (the old Lampsacus), where fell that wonderful Meteoric Stone in the 58th Olympiad; described by Aristotle, Plutarch, and Pliny; and by the latter two writers affirmed to be still seen in the place where it fell. Its great size, and other physical marks denoted, point to the possibility of its being yet discovered by intelligent research on the spot. Though the presumption comes next to certainty, there would be interest in knowing by actual analysis, that an Aerolite, thus authenticated in its antiquity, contains the same material elements as those reaching the Earth in our own day. It would add to the many evidences of the physical identity of those material elements pervading space, out of which, under the operation of higher laws than we can yet comprehend, our Solar System has been moulded into its present form and order. The theory of Laplace is ever deriving fresh verification as science advances in new paths of progress.

On my first visit to Cincinnati, in 1856, when returning from St. Louis and the Western States, I resided at the Observatory on Mount Adams with the family of my friend Professor Mitchell, whose reputation as an observer, as well as popular writer on Astronomy, is well established. The spot is one magnificent in position, almost overhanging the great City so recently created, and overlooking for a distance of more than twenty miles the beautiful valley of the Ohio—that noble river which has called Cincinnati into life and prosperity. The great Achromatic telescope, which the zeal of Mr. Mitchell obtained for this Observatory (also the workmanship of Bavaria), ranked then as second in America. The nights I passed here, under a sky of intense clearness, afforded me the finest views of the Nebulæ and Double Stars I have ever enjoyed—views before which all earthly landscape becomes insignificant. On one of these nights we were strangely interrupted by three fires breaking out in the City underneath, spreading rapidly as they do in newly-built American towns, and veiling with a cloud of earthly smoke the wonders of the heaven above.

I found much also to gratify me here in Mr. Mitchell's inventions for giving exactness to his record of observations, by aid of electricity as well as by his own mechanical devices—striking examples of the aid which each science renders to others, seemingly the most remote. His Memoir on ' Personal Equations,' founded on differences in the individual faculty of observation, is an able account of a very remarkable phenomenon; fully confirmed, and enlarged in all its details by the tabular results as to ' Personality in Observation' obtained at Greenwich and elsewhere. What I had myself written on the ' Mental Functions in their Relation to Time' rendered the matter of this Memoir very interesting to me. It is a subject which has been strikingly illustrated by the researches of Helmholz and others ' On Time, as concerned in the Transmission of Volition and Sensation through the Nerves :' researches among the most interesting and important of modern Physiology, and valuable as another example of those recent methods of experiment which make the discoveries in one branch of science the agents and interpreters in the prosecution of another. For here, again, that wonderful element of Electricity was the chief agent in research—a mystery to us still in its own nature, yet, more than any other elementary power, aiding in the solution of the mysteries which confront us elsewhere in the world of nature.*

At the time when I visited these several Observatories Astronomy had not entered into that new phase of discoveries which have given fresh lustre to a Science

---

* On the outbreak of the late Civil War, my friend Professor Mitchell quitted the Observatory at Albany, to which he had been appointed, and entered the Federal Army. His habitual ardour and zeal, testified in various enterprises, speedily raised him to the rank of General. He did not, however, live to see the end of the struggle. The fever of the Carolina coast was fatal to him, as to so many other brave men.

already marvellous in its record of human attainments. To the knowledge of celestial distances, magnitudes, motions and mutual perturbations, extending far beyond our own system, has now been added a knowledge of the material elements existing in the Sun ; and in many of those more remote Suns, whose Light, despite its inconceivable velocity, takes years of passage through space to reach us. Of the total number of elementary substances known on our globe, nearly one-fourth have been discovered in the solar photosphere ; and by methods of discovery next to mathematical in evidence, and forming in themselves a new branch of science. They establish conclusions of vast import to all our conceptions of the Universe, in teaching the unity of that Power which acted in the creation of worlds. These high advancements of human knowledge, though yet belonging to a few only, strikingly attest the wonderful faculties bestowed on Man by his Creator, and their capacity for still larger attainments in the future.

While speaking on Astronomy, I am tempted to notice a spectacle, having a certain association with this science, which I do not remember to have seen recorded either in prose or poetry, though well meriting description in either way. This spectacle requires, however, a combination of circumstances rarely occurring — a perfectly clear Eastern and Western horizon, and an entirely level intervening surface, such as that of the Sea or the African desert—the former rendering the illusion, if such it may be called, most complete to the eye. The view I seek to describe embraces the orb of the

setting Sun, and that of the full Moon rising in the East
—*both above the horizon at the same time.* The spectator
on the Sea between, if he can discard from mental vision
the vessel on which he stands, and regard only these two
great globes of Heaven and the Sea-horizon circling
unbroken around him, gains a conception through this
spectacle, clearer than any other conjunction can give,
of those wonderful relations which it is the triumph of
Astronomy to disclose. All objects are excluded save
the Sun, the Moon, and our own Globe between; but
these objects are such in themselves that their very
simplicity and paucity of number enhances the sense
of the sublime. Only twice or thrice, however, have I
witnessed the sight in its completeness—once on a
Mediterranean voyage between Minorca and Sardinia—
once in crossing the desert from Suez to Cairo, when
the same full Moon showed me, a few hours later, the
very different but picturesque sight of one of the annual
caravans of Mecca pilgrims, with a long train of camels,
making their night march towards the Red Sea. Such
memories cling to the mind, while those of much later
events are often lost in the current of time.

I have before mentioned Geology as a science of early
interest to me; and, though my method of travel has
prevented any exact research, the mere roadside observation of rocks has had its pleasures and advantages.
Here indeed the railroad, injurious to observation in
many ways, tells the traveller by its deep cuttings and
sharp sections of strata, something more of the country
through which he is passing than could be learnt on the

old carriage roads. On every occasion, where possible, I have sought access to Mines. Beginning in youth with the Northumberland Collieries and Cheshire Salt mines, I have subsequently visited the Copper and Tin mines of Cornwall; the Salt mines of Austria and Galicia; the Copper and Silver mines of the Hartz Mountains; the Copper and Iron mines of Sweden; the Coal and Iron mines of Pennsylvania; the Mineral Pitch mines of Albania; and the Lead mines of Murcia in Spain, where the evidences are seen of workings of far older date, stretching back, it may be, to those Phœnician and Carthaginian times which still furnish so many unsolved problems to history.

At Andreasberg, in the Hartz Mountains, I descended to a considerable depth the Sampson Mine; the workings of which, at the extreme depth of 2,450 feet, were then, and possibly still are, the deepest on the surface of the globe, though not so near to its centre as some of our English Coal mines in Durham and Lancashire. To the latter we must look for evidence of the depth to which the workings of Man in mines may possibly or safely be carried—a matter obviously of high concernment to the future industry and wealth of England, and offering many curious problems for practical science to solve. Is it too much to hope that science may hereafter disclose new sources of mechanical or motive power, thereby sparing those on which we now chiefly depend? I have elsewhere alluded to the tides of seas and rivers, as a power capable of larger and more various application than we have yet given to it. May we not say the same of Solar heat—that great element so profusely poured upon the earth, and capable, if modern doctrines speak truly, of being stored up for ages in the vegetable organisations to which it has ministered life and growth ? Admitting this interpretation of facts,—which however can hardly yet be regarded as final,—may we not arrive hereafter at some method of *saving*, or *storing up* for present or prospective use, a portion of that vast super-fluity of heat which the solar beams periodically supply, and which, as far as we know, is lost again in outer space ? It is enough here to put these questions. The future alone can answer them.

My subterranean travels have included Caves also. I visited in 1860 the Mammoth Cave of Kentucky ; less striking in the beauty of its calcareous stalactites than that of Adelsberg ; but astonishing in its extent, and the magnitude of its rock-vaults and subterranean rivers —forming altogether the most wonderful, yet known, of these great *cracks* or *erosions* of the crust of the earth ; and surrounded, moreover, by a forest scenery which alone might invite a traveller to the spot. . . . Four years later I accompanied those eminent naturalists, Dr. Falconer and Mr. Busk (the former unhappily now no more) in their examination of the remarkable Caves and Rifts at Gibraltar ; opened out to research by the zealous labours of Captain Broom, and adding fresh proof of the chronological connection of Man with animal species now extinct, and with periods of time anterior to the latest revolutions of the earth's surface. The results derived from the limited localities hitherto examined in this new path of enquiry, give good augury of what may be expected from similar research in other and more distant regions of the globe. Such research, indeed, is now unceasingly pressed onwards by its connection with all the most important questions in natural history under present examination. Strange it is that even these more recent remains, and the innumerable vestiges of far older worlds of life, should have been so totally hidden from or misinterpreted by man, until it came to our day to discover and decipher them! The present century of physical science, almost burdened by its weight of discoveries, might well be designated to posterity by this act of progress alone.

In other branches of physics less connected with travel, I have endeavoured, as already stated, to keep up with the current—certain that, if loitering behind, it would be difficult or impossible to regain it. Mere reading on these subjects, or desultory occasions of taking them up, are very far from sufficient to fulfil this object. That present interblending of the physical sciences which facilitates and is so fruitful of discovery, becomes an impediment to those who seek access to them cursorily, or from one side only. As regards myself, I have been much aided in my object by a constant intercourse maintained with the men most eminent in active research; and by being present, whenever it was possible, at all experiments denoting discovery in progress or actually accomplished. What is thus learnt by the eye is far more firmly fixed in the mind than by any other mode of instruction. A single experiment will often thoroughly teach what no description, however elaborate, can convey to the understanding.

My connection with the Royal Institution has here been very valuable to me. A long and intimate friendship with Faraday, succeeding to that with Young and Davy, kept me in the train of those great discoveries which have illustrated their names, and given a well-merited fame to the place in which they were made. Like the observatory of the astronomer, the laboratory of the experimental philosopher is, or ought to be, a spot set apart from the turmoil of the world without. I have often felt a certain emotion in coming suddenly from the crowded and noisy pavements of Piccadilly to those silent laboratories in Albemarle Street (almost buried below ground); where science, working through fruitful experiment, has disclosed so many secrets of the natural world. It is in some respects even a more striking contrast than any of those I have denoted in my life of travel.

Some of Faraday's researches, and especially those on Diamagnetism and the Magnetisation of Light, I sought, through an article in the 'Quarterly Review,' to make known somewhat beyond that pale which usually limits to a few the knowledge and full appreciation of such discoveries.* With the same motive, at a later time and applied to other topics, I wrote one or two articles on Modern Chemistry and its relations to the Atomic Theory—a subject which now embraces,

---

* A very interesting letter from Faraday gave me the assurance that I had rightly interpreted his discoveries in the article mentioned above.

directly or indirectly, the whole philosophy of the material world ; and brings us into contact, through the reciprocal relations of Matter and Force, with the most profound problems that can come before the mind of man.

A friend of mine, equally eminent in public life and literary accomplishments, strikingly expressed to me a short time ago, his feeling of passing into another world when the physical discoveries of the present day were casually presented to him. His own power of mind enabled him to look some way into this new world, and to appreciate what human genius and labour have accomplished within it. But, generally speaking, a hard line of demarcation—depending often indeed on mental temperament — is interposed between these respective fields of literature and science. My own recollection furnishes me with only three or four instances—Young and Herschel amongst them—where eminence has been attained by the same individual in each. The instances are far more frequent where the wonders of the natural world, and the wondrous methods employed in their research, remain utterly unknown to minds of high endowment in other parts of human knowledge. As I have remarked elsewhere, however, this barrier is gradually giving way. The discoveries and speculations of modern science have made so deep an inroad on prior opinions, as well as on all the conditions of human life, that a certain amount of such knowledge is forced even upon those most unwilling to accept the changes going on.

CHAPTER XII.

I COME now to one of the few subjects which still remain to me before closing this Narrative. An author always seeks to give, or to obtain from others, some sort of record of what he has written ; and, though not making any large claim for myself in this capacity, my writings may perhaps justify an enumeration of them, with some slight explanatory comment on a few of the number, especially those which concern Medicine and Mental Physiology.

I have already spoken of my earliest work (if indeed it can rightly be called mine), the 'Agricultural Survey of Cheshire ;' and of the Introduction and Chapters on Icelandic History and Literature, contributed to Sir George Mackenzie's narrative of our travels in Iceland in 1810. I have mentioned also the volumes relating my 'Travels in Albania, Thessaly, and Greece,' which, as well as that on Iceland, went through two editions. This work would have been more valuable, as regards the Albanian portion of my journeys in Turkey, but for that robbery of many of my papers to which allusion has elsewhere been made. I have also in a former place spoken of the numerous articles contributed to the Edinburgh and Quarterly Reviews, chiefly on scientific subjects, and written for the most part during my autumnal travels; giving me pleasant and salutary occupation in places and at times when I should otherwise have been harassed by a sense of loneliness. These articles, with the exception of one written during my West Indian voyage in 1870, have been discontinued for several years past ; my journeys being now much less exposed to the chances of misadventure, and generally made with some companionship of travel.* A certain number of the Essays were collected, and published five or six years ago in a separate volume, of which a second edition came out a few months afterwards, and subsequently a very able German translation. Short though the interval was between these editions, it embraced several fresh discoveries needing to be recorded. It is difficult, indeed, in these days to frame a scientific history, with the chance of its having other permanent value than as a record of the changes continually in progress. A work on Modern Chemistry, for instance, is antiquated before ten years have gone by—antiquated even in nomenclature and theory ; still more so as a record of the actual acquirements of the science. Astronomy might seem to promise greater stability; yet, as I have just stated, every year teems with fresh discoveries in our own Sun and Solar System, and in the Suns and Sidereal Universe beyond—discoveries which

---

* This article (*Edinburgh Review*, January 1871), based on the remarkable treatises of M. Langel, was in effect a review of the state and speculations of modern science, in relation to the great problems which Matter, Force, Life, Electricity, &c., bring before us.

may well amaze even those who have given their lives to this great study.

I might say yet more of the pleasure and advantage I have derived from writing the articles to which I am alluding. Unfettered as to time and subjects, and having no other motive for writing than the occupation itself, this occupation became an amusement rather than a labour ; and profitable, whenever science was concerned, by better defining to my own mind whatever knowledge I happened to possess on the subject. Though writing solely for the two great political Reviews, I doubt whether a single political opinion or feeling would be found in what I have contributed to their pages.

Reviewing myself as a Reviewer (a somewhat unusual thing to do), I can honestly say that I have ever sought to be fair and impartial ; with an inclination, it may be from temperament, to use the critical pen very gently. This disposition was favoured by the nature of the subjects I usually adopted for my articles, as well as by the places in which I wrote most of them, far removed from the critical atmosphere of London life. I may fairly affirm that I never composed an article under any other influence than that of the subject ; and except in two instances—one of these the review of the 'Cosmos' of Humboldt, already mentioned, and the other of trifling import—I have never been made aware of any offence given by what I have written. I venture to believe that few writers of more than twenty articles in Reviews could make the same assertion. I have pleasure in making it.

The first edition of my 'Medical Notes and Reflections,' the work of which I desire to speak somewhat more in detail, was published in 1839; the third and last edition in 1855. A good German translation of it by Dr. Wallach appeared soon after. Its plan, as a series of detached Essays recording my experience on various subjects of pathology and practice, was in some sort made necessary by the fact of my never having been attached to a Hospital—a condition requisite for that complete study of particular disease, which such institutions alone can afford. Other medical works had before been composed on the same plan.

With some advantages, it has this serious drawback, that, from the several subjects having no indication in the title of the volume (and Titles have now become a matter of artistic elaboration), the Essays, even if read, cannot easily be recollected or referred to by those entering upon the same track of enquiry. I have experienced this in various instances as regards the volume in question, and in one or two instances have been somewhat mortified in finding certain of my views adopted in other works, under ignorance of their having been discussed before.

Nevertheless, I have much reason to be satisfied with the success of this work, and indulge the belief that it has aided in establishing several conclusions of practical value. I would allude here especially to Chapters XXII. and XXIII., in which are discussed two very important points of practice, the subjects of much controversy, and still not free from conflict of opinion.*   On these points what occurred to me in the early part of my professional life as *questions*, were matured by further experience into *convictions ;* and these convictions I have sought to express as strongly as I felt to be due to their practical value.   The changes which have actually occurred in this direction, whencesoever derived, are well worthy of being noted in the recent history of Physic. They suggest reflections applying to the future as well as to the past, and involving deeply the character of Medicine as a science.

In other Chapters of this Volume, especially in the last Edition, I have endeavoured to give weight and currency to certain parts of practice, collateral, it may be said, to those just named.   These suggestions are founded on the conviction, also the fruit of experience, that many conditions described and treated as disease are natural actions, set up and tending to obviate or remove some existing cause of disorder in the system ; and that the interruption of such actions is not merely needless, but often mischievous in effect.   It is a maxim of very old medical authority, that where Nature is at

---

* These Chapters are entitled *On the Abuse of Purgative Medicines*, and *On Bleeding in Affections of the Brain*—both matters of obvious importance, and the latter especially the subject of various opinion and controversy, in its connection with the general change as to blood-letting in medical prac-tice.   This change has become such in extent that, unless justified by some radical alteration in the national temperament—and I know no collateral evidence of this—the suspicion must remain, either that we are now erring by default on the one side, or that there has been for a long period an injurious excess on the other.   The experience and judgment of the physician are continually called upon to face this question, which is such in its practical importance that it cannot rightly be left in abeyance.

work in her own way, we are bound not to check or meddle with her operations. This in truth is well known as one of the oldest questions in medical practice, and needing the highest qualities of discrimination in the practitioner, not merely for the sake of science, but as a matter pertaining to professional credit and public welfare. In Chapter XVII., under the title of 'Internal Hemorrhages, and Morbid Secretions as the Subjects of Medical Treatment,' I have introduced some particular examples illustrating this principle, and themselves very important as questions of practice. But more remains to be done, and will assuredly be accomplished, in this direction of progress. It is one of the safest paths for the physician to pursue, when seeking for some general principle of practice, to which this may be subordinate.

In another Chapter of this Volume 'On Diseases commonly occurring but once in Life,' I have dealt with a subject of deep interest, but as obscure as interesting. The great problem it involves has not yet been reached even by approximation. Expressing it by a single question—What is that change in a living body which gives exemption from a certain disease for the remainder of life, when the individual has once gone through it?—or yet more specifically—In what physical conditions does A, having had the small-pox or been vaccinated, differ from himself before such protection was given, or from B, who has never obtained it? This question, yet unsolved, includes within itself many collateral problems, the legitimate objects of future research. Here, as in so many other cases in physical science, a single door fairly opened would give access to numerous secrets of nature, inaccessible by other approach. In seeking to open it, one main fact must be kept in mind, viz. that all the diseases thus characterised are *contagious* in kind. This consideration is obviously essential to any true theory of the phenomena ; and it has the greater value, in my view of the subject, from bringing in Life, under some form or other, as the element concerned in giving contagious character to these diseases and defining their course. Fully admitting our ignorance as to all such subtle phenomena, I am unable to conceive any explanation from which this element can be excluded.*

In other Chapters, and generally throughout the Volume, I have sought to draw more attention than is usually given to those collateral remedies, mental as well as bodily, which have often a far higher value than the drugs crowding and perplexing our Pharmacopœias. Here again the oldest masters of Medicine, and Hippocrates especially, might largely be quoted. But the topic is one that needs not the authority of any prior age,

* Few can conceive, or admit these conditions of life, utterly imperceptible by any of our senses—a difficulty very intelligible under ignorance of what the microscope has done in revealing living organic forms, to which the unaided eye finds no access. But the microscope tells a feeble tale, compared with the proofs furnished by higher physical researches, of a divisibility of matter, whether living or lifeless, which figures fail adequately to express. The term Infinite, a shadow to our reason in every case, is valueless when we apply it to those atoms and molecules the actions and changes of which form the subjects of all science, and which, inconceivably minute though they be, yet in their aggregated energies give origin to the grandest phenomena of the Universe.

resting as it ought to do upon the common-sense of all mankind; and requiring only that this common-sense should be rescued from the fetters which fashion or technical forms impose upon it. The prescription of the physician, however learned in its Latin and pharmacy, is but a slender part of his professional duty. Of far greater import generally to the patient is his watchfulness over the economy of the sick chamber — its temperature, ventilation, cleanliness, and quiet—the various appliances, even of changes of posture, fitted to relieve pain and procure rest—all too that the *lenis sermo* and *hilaris vultus* (I willingly quote from Celsus) can justifiably do in soothing and giving hope. A dry and technical rule of practice ill compensates for the absence of these simpler and happier ministrations.*

Much more might be said on this subject were it within my present scope. I willingly admit that greater attention is now given to these points than was the case when I began my professional life, and never without ample evidence of good thus gained. But there is still great room for improvement, and especially among

---

* Various passages might be quoted from the ancient medical authors showing how much value they attached to these minutiæ of practice, even as regards the outward demeanour of the physician. These writings well deserve more general reading and attention than is now given to them. Who now ever looks at Aretæus?—a writer of beautiful Ionic Greek, and as a physician full of intelligence and just discrimination. The work of Celsus abounds in practical maxims, many of which might beneficially be brought into present application. My excellent friend, Bishop Blomfield, had a high appreciation of certain parts of the writings of Hippocrates; and I believe I still possess some short extracts from them which he sent to me, written beautifully, as he always wrote the Greek characters. It was the touch of an artistic pen, and he had a certain pride in it.

those young in practice ; who, coming from the formal instruction of books, lectures, and examinations, rest too much on old names and old opinions, and lack that better learning which experience alone can give. The *nimia diligentia medici* is a phrase which especially applies to those new in the art of treating disease. It has the same practical meaning as the *trop de zèle*, against which a young diplomatist was cautioned by one of riper and more astute experience.

The Volume of which I am speaking has been thought by some to be too sceptical on points both of medical doctrine and practice. Freely admitting this tendency, which perhaps is inherent in my nature, I have sought to justify it here, not solely in particular instances, but more generally in a Chapter in which are discussed the principles of Medical Evidence—a subject well deserving to be more distinctly inculcated than it is, as an essential part of medical education ; the more especially as it is the young practitioner who most suffers from not comprehending its importance. Rightly to understand the peculiarities and difficulties of this evidence is indeed next to a necessity for the true physician. I have seen so much in my own time of crude novelties in medicine, eagerly adopted on the shallowest proof and rapidly succeeding one another in popular fashion, injuriously alike to the profession and the public, that remonstrance becomes a duty where there is even a chance of good to be obtained from it.

The sole remedy, as far as I can see, for this and other evils is to be found in a better appreciation of that evidence which really establishes medical truth. To inculcate distrust is hardly a pleasant office, but it is often wholesome or necessary; and such is the case with many of the tenets handed down to us by our fathers in medicine, as well as with the various novelties of opinion and practice growing up successively in our own time. There is a curious incapacity in some men's minds for comprehending evidence at all; a desultory love of change, whatever its shape, governs others; while we are forced to admit worldly interests as a further cause concerned in these professional aberrations. Despite all such obstacles it is well to believe, and I do believe, that much will be done to ennoble Medicine in the future, and to give it closer relation to the exact sciences. And though, in progress to this point, something must be abandoned of the pretensions hitherto assumed, and many errors put aside, this exclusion of the false or unreal is a gain to all the higher interests and duties of a physician's life.

After fifty years of practice in London, I might, and perhaps not without some justification, say a good deal more regarding the present state of the Medical Profession here, the changes it has undergone within my time, as well as the probable source and sequel of these changes. But the topic is too large, and too difficult and delicate of handling to tempt me into such digression. It is one not to be dealt with by a few curt and dogmatical phrases, whatever their import. And, further than this, the peculiarity of my own professional life, as unconnected with any of the great Hospitals of the metropolis, and limited very much to one district of London, would justly render doubtful any conclusions I might hazard on the subject. If other excuse were needful, it might be found in the numerous schemes of Medical Reform which have been suggested and partially adopted within the last twenty years—the work chiefly of the Profession itself; but under difficulties, from diversity of interests and other causes, which have hitherto prevented any satisfactory result.

But there may be more justification for a brief allusion here to those many *Charlataneries* I have witnessed in my professional career; coming rapidly in succession to one another; and each drawing largely for a time on public credulity. The name of physical science wrongly usurped, and the claim of curing every disease —a claim which carries its own refutation with it—are brought in to sanction what is purely imposture. Here, unfortunately, the tests of truth are of a kind easily overridden by extravagant pretensions, commonplace fallacies, or the strong seduction of novelty; and the particular folly or fraud is often corrected only by the intervention of some other deserving a like fate. Argument is seldom of much avail with those thus imposed upon; and the time and temper of the physician are both grievously wasted, if submitted to controversies utterly useless, where ignorant asseveration takes the place of that evidence which alone can establish a medical truth. In such cases I have myself generally found the refusal of discussion a more effectual answer than any train of reasoning. One of the sharpest

weapons in argument is Silence ; and the most provoking
to an adversary, if this were an admissible motive. But
there are few who have patience and discretion enough
to make the proper use of this resource when the
feelings, as well as reason, are called into play.*

These topics however lie beyond my present scope,
and I shall not do more than thus cursorily advert to
them. They belong in fact not to Medicine exclusively, but to human nature itself and to the history of
social life. Lord Bacon says well, ' In all superstitions
wise men follow fools : ' and this remark is strangely
justified by the hold such delusions (especially when
cloaked under a flimsy garb of science) often obtain
over the minds of men of the soundest judgment in
other matters. It is indeed a fact of common observation, that a mind strictly logical on many points, may be
weakly illogical on others ; where the seductions of
novelty and mystery come in to blind the reason. The
general conclusion is forced upon us that as long as
folly and credulity exist in the world, there is sure to
be imposture to foster and feed upon them. In another
pithy sentence of Lord Bacon, ' Men mark the hits and
not the misses,' we have an apt explanation of the
success of some of those supernatural pretensions which
have been put forward in our own day—strictly supernatural, were they true, since no definition of miracle
could exclude them from being thus denominated. In
recording as facts what would be actual suspensions of

---

* Τῆς σιγῆς βάρος is the phrase of a great Greek poet ; who nevertheless
pleaded his own cause in an Athenian court of law at the age of ninety.

the great laws of the material world, they bring in the Divine Power, as acting immediately in every such manifestation. It might be supposed that the frivolous or even vulgar character of many of these exhibitions would have exposed their true character. But they have found a partial shelter under the real mysteries of Man's nature —the phenomena of sleep and dreams, of delirium, and the many morbid or anomalous states of the brain and nervous system. To these phenomena, indeed, we may best look for explanation of many of the more innocent delusions of which I am now speaking. Familiar to us, and disregarded in ordinary life, they take fresh hold on the mind when presented under new names, and cloaked by the artifices imposed upon them.

It is curious to note how periodical these epidemic visitations of miracle have become. Mesmeric visions and prophecies, clairvoyance, spirit-rappings, table-turnings and liftings, &c., succeed one another in popular fashion ; with certain intervals between, to allow prior detections to be forgotten, and to catch the credulous of a new generation.* The reason disappears when the imagination is thus called into play. It was a shrewd observer of the foibles of the world who said that ' Folly is like matter, and cannot be annihilated.' Ancient and

---

* When stories of this kind are offered to my belief, I generally meet them by silence rather than argument. Or, if infringing upon this rule, it is by simply enquiring Whether anything has been paid at the door or elsewhere for the miracles performed ?'—leaving the inference in such case to be drawn by those who have witnessed the performance. This question does not apply to all these exhibitions; but to a certain number of them, equally credited as the others, it may very pertinently be put.

mediæval history give us the repeated record of similar delusions, the names and forms alone changed. They tend especially to fill up those gaps of time when there are no events in progress to catch the imagination, or satisfy the appetite for novelty ever present in the world. The future will doubtless be productive of them as the past has been, for they are founded on a common weakness of our nature.*

Though the greater part of my Volume of 'Medical Notes' has concern with pathology or practice, I have given one Chapter to an hypothesis, which fully satisfies my own mind, regarding the nature and manner of diffusion of the Indian Cholera. Having studied with much interest and some care the history of this extraordinary disease, in its successive epidemic forms and modes of migration over the earth, I have arrived at the conviction that its phenomena can no otherwise be explained than by looking to organic life, animal or vegetable (more probably, as I think, the former), as the source—the actual *virus*, which, *reproducing itself* (a point essential to the argument), gives origin, diffusion, and direction to the disease under the different conditions it assumes. The grounds of this conclusion I have fully stated in the Chapter referred to ; nor do I myself see how they can be impugned. The pathology of Cholera, variously disputed even under our large

* Shakespeare, to whom no side of human nature was unknown, puts into the mouths of Volscian lacqueys (Coriolanus, act iv. s. 6), a humorous picture, with much of truth in it, of the tendency of peace to evolve various follies, impostures, and even vices, which are suspended under the higher excitements of war.

experience of the disease, is not directly concerned in the argument, save as respects the limitation of the disorder to man, and the close analogy thereby furnished to those strange parasitical diseases or blights which living swarms, recognised as such, inflict upon particular species both in the vegetable and animal world.   Such analogy is not less complete in the exceptions and ano-malies than in the ordinary phenomena of these several migrating diseases.   The detailed history of this migra-tion in the case of the Indian Cholera—and a very remarkable history it is—affords in my mind the most conclusive proof of the view I have adopted; and is connected moreover with some of the most curious problems which life, under its innumerable forms, presents to our speculation.*

In the first Editions of my 'Medical Notes' there were a few Chapters having closer relation to Mental Philosophy than to Medicine.   These I removed from the last Edition, and embodied them with three or four other Essays on kindred subjects, in a small volume.

---

* This hypothesis stops short of the minute pathology of Cholera, and offers no suggestion as to treatment—a failure that belongs alike to every other view of the causes of the disease.   The duration of the epi-demic in its distinct form, in any given spot, is generally from six to eight weeks.   As long as the proportion of deaths to those attacked during this time remains the same, whatever the locality and whatever the mode of treatment (and I think I may affirm this to be so), we are compelled to admit that no valid remedy, general or specific, has yet been found.   The recoveries, more frequent as the disease is approaching its close in any given place, prove rather the lessened intensity of the virus, than the increased efficacy of the treatment, whatever this may be.   In truth the very diversity of the remedies, propounded with equal pretensions of success, becomes in itself a cogent argument that no true specific has been discovered, either wholly preventive, or curative of the disease.

entitled 'Chapters on Mental Physiology,' of which work there have been two editions. The parts of this Volume to which I attach most interest are the Chapters 'On Mental Consciousness in its Relation to Time and Succession,' and that 'On Time as an Element in Mental Functions.' In these Chapters, closely connected in argument, I have adopted a method of studying the functions of Mind, hitherto only rarely and partially employed; but capable, as I think, of eliciting many facts which other methods fail to reach, and of explaining some of those anomalies which perplex our systems of Psychology. This subject indeed is too vast and complex to be approached from any single point, or comprised within any one scheme. And, above all, it requires to be freed from that 'contexture of words' which so often puts impediments in the way of truth, especially where the mental functions are concerned. The single word *consciousness*, for instance, simple as it may seem, and essential as an exponent of these functions, is nevertheless a term of doubtful and disputed meaning, when applied to those mixed bodily and mental phenomena which make up the totality of Life. It is differently defined by different writers; a diversity indeed not less manifest in numerous other terms which have played their part in the metaphysics of all ages.

There is another Chapter in this Volume, entitled 'On the Brain as a Double Organ,' which I may notice, not only from the many curious and difficult questions it involves, but also from its having produced the dedication to me of a volume by a learned and ingenious man, Dr. Wigan, since deceased. Under the somewhat startling title of the ' Duality of Mind,' Dr. Wigan stretches his own conclusions far beyond my more limited view. He affirms that I have opened a path, and been on the verge of a great discovery, without attaining a truth which was fairly within my reach. The discovery of the Duality of Mind he claims for himself; seeking to justify his invasion of *personal identity* by the many strange cases known to every physician, where a curiously marked *duplicity*—or what, to avoid ambiguity, I may call *contradiction*—occurs in the consciousness, the moral feelings, and the will of the same individual, at the same time, or in such close mutual sequence as to give the aspect of being so. In a former part of this Memoir, when relating the projected attempt on Mr. Canning's life, I furnished one striking instance in point. Others, as extraordinary, I have given in the Essay alluded to above ; and my experience has since brought before me cases still more strange in the frequent and sudden alternation of states of mind as alien to one another as mania and the most perfect sanity ; without obvious cause, and with entire unconsciousness of the individual of the changes thus occurring. The latter fact, that of unconsciousness, often occurring in analogous cases, is as mysterious as are the occurrences themselves. Without accepting any such theory as that of the Duality of Mind for their solution, it may well be admitted that these phenomena form a very perplexing chapter, and painful as well as perplexing, in the history of this portion of our nature.

CHAPTER XIII.

THIS is all I need say regarding my connection with the Press ; which, though unambitious in its pretensions, has not, I hope, been without its practical uses. There is little probability of my ever publishing again ; but I shall leave behind me a large volume of manuscript papers, consigned to the care of my Sons, to deal with as their judgment may suggest—well knowing that I cannot place them in better hands. These papers are, in fact, compilations from miscellaneous notes, the thoughts and speculations of former years; reduced into more definite form as regards the subjects, and studiously rendered as concise as possible. The latter point I especially mention, because many of the topics discussed are such as have been matter of controversy for ages ; thereby becoming entangled in a network of vague words, and of arguments which, though novel in aspect, are in reality only new facings to old opinions. What has been well called ' the art of talking unintelligibly on matters of which we are ignorant,' belongs so especially to some of these topics, that in dealing with them I have sought above all things to distinguish between what is *known*, and what is *not known ;*—and further to define as far as can be done, what, from the nature and limitations of human reason, can *never be known at all.* Brevity, attained by crucial instances, is the soul of all argument in subjects of this nature; and such for the satisfaction of my own mind I have sedulously sought to bring into all that I have written. The papers thus denoted have furnished a very agreeable as well as salutary occupation for those leisure hours which in later years have been more largely at my disposal. But to bring them together in shape and fitness for publication would require a more laborious revision than I should probably be able to bestow.

I have noted below a few of the subjects of these papers, sufficient to indicate their general character.* Some of them will be seen to involve those great questions in the physical sciences, to which so much subtle and careful experiment, profound thought, and even mathematical analysis, are now directed; with the assurance of higher attainment, whatever be the ultimate limits of research. The continuous and rapid progress of these sciences makes it certain that much of what I have written in bringing my detached notes together, will soon be superseded by the discovery of new facts, or the reduction to more general laws of those we now possess. Already indeed, certain of the speculations in

---

* Unity of Creative Power ; Plurality of Worlds ; Natural Theology ; Differences of Religious Belief ; Evil in the World ; Life on the Earth, and the Relation of Man to other Animals ; Perfectibility of Man ; Animal Instincts ; Generation, and Origin of Species ; Sleep and Dreaming ; Mental Functions in relation to Time ; Matter, Force and Motion in Physical Phenomena ; Atomic Theory ; Ether and the Electric Element.

which I have ventured to indulge have become the property of others, and been vindicated with more ability and knowledge than I could give to their illustration. So far from regretting this, I feel satisfaction in finding them endorsed by higher authority than my own, and more likely therefore to be adopted as objects of further enquiry.

I might instance here a subject which has always deeply interested me—the question, namely 'What is Electricity?'—an enquiry as subtle as the element to which it relates, and perplexed by phrases which have become the formulæ of science—necessary perhaps to expound facts, but involving hypotheses which facts themselves have hardly yet justified. The view I entertain as possible or even probable, that the Electric element is identical with the Ether of Space—variously modified in its conditions by conjunction with the grosser forms of terrestrial matter—may doubtless come under this very condemnation of want of evidence. The existence of Ether itself as a material element, admits of no other present proof than the necessity of such medium to explain phenomena in which the transmission of force or power is concerned. But where direct proof is wanting, and perhaps inaccessible, a certain amount of hypothesis may fairly be admitted; and, as far as I can see, there is no view regarding the Electrical element, yet propounded, which satisfies the general conditions of the problem better than that just stated.

Treating this subject at greater length in my manu-

script papers, I have fully expressed the difficulties of
the problem and the very general form that must be
given to any conclusion adopted.   The whole argument
hinges on the simple question whether Electricity is a
material element in itself, or merely a material action
or atomic change in the bodies evolving or conducting
the electrical state.   Vast though our knowledge is of
Electrical phenomena, and vast the command obtained
over this extraordinary power, the first letters are still
wanting to the alphabet of the science.   In some respects indeed, the difficulties of the elementary problem are even augmented with our knowledge of
phenomena.   In this instance as in many others (especially where the conception of Force enters integrally
into the question), those whose researches and thoughts
go deepest are best prepared to endorse the words of
Laplace, '*Notre ignorance est immense*,' as the expression of a truth underlying all our knowledge.   Even
where science seems most complete, as in that great
law of Gravitation which has told the existence and
place of a new planet from the perturbations of one
before known, there is always an unanswered question
beneath—'What is Gravitation itself?'—a question
which, like that of—What is Electricity? remains for
some higher and happier conception in the time to
come.*   Faraday—a hint from whose genius has often

---

* While speaking of Electricity, let me briefly record the impression—I
might almost say *emotion*—I have felt in my later voyages to and from
America, when presumably close upon the line of the Atlantic Telegraph.
Gazing here from the ship's side on the surface of this great Ocean, with
the knowledge that at the depth of two miles underneath, there lay a cord

furnished a volume for the future—supposed as probable some connection between these two Forces. Such may hereafter be disclosed ; but the only fact at present common to both, is our ignorance of the nature of the primary powers concerned in their phenomena.

Two among my many papers still unpublished, relate to subjects already discussed in the Volume on 'Mental Physiology,' but which I have since kept always before me for thought and observation. These are the various phenomena of Sleep and Dreaming, and of Animal Instincts—topics of profound interest to men who think or observe at all ; and bringing us into closest contact with those mysterious relations of mental and bodily life which form at once the foundation and the crucial problems of all physiology. While admitting the value of much that has been written on these subjects, I by no means think they have been exhausted to our research. The former especially—those wonderful phenomena of Sleep and Dreams which occupy nearly a third part of human life, yet are lost to our reason from their very familiarity—may be treated, as I believe, by a method of enquiry more prolific of results than any hitherto adopted. This method I have followed both in the published Essay and in that which I have by me ; but with various

of Wires stretching from the Old to the New World—wires not inert, but transmitting an invisible agent, the messenger of man, with a velocity of which Lightning is the fit expression, since Lightning itself is the messenger —these things, thought of at the moment, may well move the mind to a mixed feeling of wonder and awe. We are here contemplating the greatest triumph of Man, in the dominion thus obtained over one of the most powerful and mysterious of the Forces in the Universe around him.

enlargements upon it in the latter, founded on closer and more continuous observation. Such observation on dreams, however, is not so easy as it may seem. These ' children of an idle brain ' cannot be readily brought to give evidence of themselves and their vagaries, exact enough to satisfy what science requires for their full elucidation.*

The other subject, that of Animal Instincts, is one of deep interest in itself, and yet more so in its inseparable connection with those profound problems of the development and diversity of Life and Organisation, which are now awaiting solution, if indeed capable of being solved. It is a research in which, though furnished with innumerable facts and instances, we have never, either by reason or speculation, got beyond the threshold of that question of *Origin*, which applies alike to all. Whatever be the final limit to research, the paths of present enquiry are well marked out. These have in view mainly, the hereditary nature of Instincts—their relations to structure and structural changes—their connection with habits and casual conditions of life—and the influences upon them of Reason and the Will in the higher grades of creation. Even in this slight statement it will be seen how wide is the field for further

---

* I have quoted here one of those happy phrases which few but Shakespeare could have coined. The whole passage indeed in which Mab comes before us as the Queen of Dreams is one which no other poet could have written. It gives a sort of longing for the restoration of some of those harmless superstitions which amused and beguiled the vacant hours of English provincial life. Selden laments the loss of these even in his day : ' There never was a merry world since the fairies left dancing and the parsons left conjuring.'

research, both by observation and experiment. What I have written on the subject has been directed chiefly to indicate the objects, methods, and presumable limits of such research—the latter consideration qualified by keeping in view the many cases in physical science where what were once deemed insuperable barriers, have been either broken down or circuitously evaded and passed by.

Whether any of these manuscripts will be published in my lifetime is very uncertain—according to my present views, probably not. They would indeed, in any case, need thorough revision, seeing how much has since been written on most of the topics concerned. But I may again well say that they have yielded me much pleasant occupation in the act of bringing my scattered thoughts and notes together—a valuable result to myself, whatever may become of them. They have had a further and more important use, in better defining my own ideas on points which have ever been the subject of controversy and verbal disputation. An old author says : 'Discourse makes notions limpid and just.' Writing serves yet better, as my experience tells me, to the same end. It gives closer *correlation* (borrowing a word now become of familiar use) to the thoughts or theories which have passed through the mind at different times ; in which errors are often detected by their being thus brought under the coercion and correction of the pen.

I shall probably then still indulge myself in what I find to be a recreation of life ; with very careful watching for that time, certain to arrive, when the thoughts as well as the outward senses become dimmed by age. Le Sage's admirable tale of the Archbishop's Homily has not been lost upon me. The detection of incompetence indeed, as far as scientific subjects are concerned, is rendered more easy by the very nature of the subjects themselves. The intellect, when faltering from age or other cause, finds itself speedily checked if seeking to encounter such topics as the inter-relations of Matter and Force ; the Atomic systems of Chemistry ; the Spectrum Analysis ; the several theories of Ether and Electricity ; and the many similar problems which engage and agitate the scientific philosophy of our day. Even in its full maturity of power, the mind is often forced to halt in face of these great questions, gathering up strength for fresh encounter with them. Age does not readily repair itself for such encounters.

No one indeed can have studied physiology without learning the limits of intellectual labour, and the other various signs which mark the modes and degrees of mental decay. In a former part of this Narrative, when speaking of that remarkable man Dr. Wollaston, I mentioned the minute observation he directed to his own waning faculties—testing by experiments upon himself the gradual changes produced by cerebral disease. But, apart from all disease, there are those inevitable changes which enter into the very definition of old age, and have been the theme of philosophers and poets as well as the common adages of mankind. The expectant watch for these I have of late years exercised in my own case; and not without various detection of their occurrence—thus far, I believe I may say, chiefly in the functions of the senses and memory, those more mechanical parts of our mental nature. I will not speak of this self-examination as altogether an agreeable one, for I have had various enjoyment through life in the use of my faculties, such as they are. But I find a certain compensation in looking at these changes physiologically; and even at times some self-complacent satisfaction— however strange the avowal may seem—in noting their frequent accordance with prior opinions or speculations of my own.

In truth, the philosophy of the human mind receives few illustrations so valuable as those derived from the study of its early growth and eventual decay. Child-hood especially, in its progress from the cradle upwards, is a school in which the most learned may gain fresh knowledge. And here, as in physical science, simple and familiar facts, if duly noted, are often more instruc-tive, and the germ of greater results, than volumes of the most recondite research. In my own case, while age has been growing upon me, I have paid especial atten-tion to the phenomena of Memory and those of Sleep and Dreams—topics familiar to my reflections in other ways and at prior times of life. Long ago, indeed, I wrote a Chapter on the Memory, as it is affected by age and disease; and personal experience confirms what I then stated on observation of others. My own memory, without any marked peculiarity, was perhaps what might fairly be called a good one. Of its enfeeblement in

z

certain ways I am fully conscious, and the changes are such as accord with very general observation. The names of familiar persons and things are now frequently forgotten or not readily recalled. The mind often halts even as to common words ; and recovers them in the end, not by any effort of will, but by some sudden and almost impulsive suggestion. Recent events and dates are easily lost or pass into confusion, while those of long prior time still hold firm root and their right place in remembrance. The failures of memory just described I especially note from their practical bearing on the common concerns of the day. There are few, I believe, who do not feel conscious of such change in one degree or other. In what the altered aptitude to receive and retain impressions and ideas, consists, is one of those mysteries in the mechanism of this faculty on which we can do little more than blindly speculate.

Anomalies such as I now describe are casually incident to every time of life ; but they appertain to old age as irretrievable changes, due to causes of which no physiology can render account. While recognising them in progress in myself, as I have seen and studied them in others, I feel thankful that they are still only such in amount as to interfere little with anything important in the occupations or duties of life.* Various other changes indeed simultaneously go on, mitigating their

---

* A stray line of Menander—one of the few unhappily left to us— often occurs to me when comparing my experience of these changes in myself with my observation of it in others :—

Πρὸς ταῦθ᾽ ὁρῶν, γίνωσκε σαυτὸν ὅστις εἶ.

effect, and making an acquiescence in them more easy, as far as thought or volition have any concern in the matter.

I have taken note also of certain changes in the conditions of Sleep and Dreaming, of which my own experience of later years tells me. It is difficult, indeed, in any case to decipher the fleeting objects which belong to this land of shadows—the ἔθνος ὀνείρων—that marvellous alternation of existence which seems almost to dissever the continuity of our being. I cannot here seek to analyse or describe the changes just denoted as they occur to myself. I might however do this much more easily, through the method I have elsewhere proposed of viewing the various and strange phenomena of dreams, since they are all in accordance with it. In this place it is enough briefly to say that these changes chiefly show themselves in a less instant and perfect separation of the sleeping and waking states. The transition is consciously felt which a line of Dante finely describes, '*E pensamento in sogno transmutai.*' The mind lingers longer on the border-land between the two states—the sleep generally is less profound ; and dreams on this account are more vividly recollected, and with more difficulty dissevered from the realities the senses bring with them on awakening. Of these conditions I have continual evidence in my own case—instructive at least, if not such as rightly to be deemed amusing. A more frequent and importunate demand for sleep during the day is another fact of change—seemingly of little import, yet pointing to that condition of extreme age, when sleep usurps still more completely on waking existence, and life itself becomes little better than a chronic dream —the ῎Οναρ 'ημερόφαντον of the poet, in this very sense of application.

I am unwilling however when about to close my Narrative, to dwell longer on these more sombre topics —if I may so term what I have hitherto regarded with more curiosity than anxiety, and with a sort of *experimental* interest in devising means to obviate the effects of the changes going on. As regards the latter object, I may state one simple maxim—the more valuable because simple—not to allow the mind to be jaded and overdone by its own workings, whatever be the object to which these are directed. Fatigue of the intellectual faculties is always, more or less, an impairment of their vital power—reparable by repose in common cases, but becoming a fixed impairment if habitually repeated. The word *fatigue* indeed is often misappropriated to what might more fitly be called indolence—itself an injury to the faculties by their disuse. To this of course I do not here allude ; nor to those real and more important cases, chiefly of early life, where the mind suffers from being forced upon work alien to its natural propensities, or above its powers. What I mainly seek to inculcate, is that which my experience tells me to be the best management of the mind under ordinary occupations at every time of life ; but very especially when old age is coming on, and the mental powers have lost their elasticity ; if indeed not subjected to more serious causes of decay.

This is the time in which to economise what remains

of life through the several faculties which constitute it—not by disuse of these faculties (a point on which I have already said enough), but by sparing them any such excess of use as to fatigue and exhaust their power. This excess is not indeed frequent in old age, except under some compulsion of circumstances of which premature old age is the unhappy result. But the rule, as I have sought to apply it to myself, includes those many minor occasions which occur in every-day life, and for this very reason needs to be more carefully observed. If the mind becomes harassed by vain attempt at recollection, I abandon the attempt. If the attention flags from drowsiness, I put aside the occupation, whatever it be. If perplexed by any matter hard to comprehend—and the objects of human science at this time, as already stated, include many such—I shun what is an injurious confusion of mind by passing away to some alien subject ; with the fair probability of better compassing the difficulty when a pause of rest or other employment has intervened. These may seem the petty instances of a commonplace wisdom ; but, nevertheless, they are worthy of attention from those who wish to make a fair struggle against decay—or, as I would rather express it, to preserve as long as can be done the faculties with which God has endowed them.

The precepts and methods directed to the preservation of the bodily powers are much more familiarly known and applied—an evidence of the greater degree in which they engage the feelings of mankind at large ; and needfully perhaps, as regards the general conditions of human life. But these precepts, though familiar, are by no means faultless. I have already noticed one or two instances of error; and, were I writing a medical or physiological treatise, I might easily add to the number. One fundamental yet very simple maxim of preservation, applies not less to the bodily than to the mental powers—that, namely, of *using* without *straining* them. The *sense of fatigue* is a test which every man has in his own hands. All habits of prior life, wholesome in themselves, may beneficially as well as safely be maintained, until *felt* to become laborious and exhausting; and then quitted, not suddenly, but by gradual adaptation to the growing infirmities of age. Such general maxims are often indeed difficult in their application to the endless contingencies and anomalies of human life; but nevertheless a wise man will keep them in mind as a guidance in questionable cases.

That I may not abuse one of the prerogatives of old age by running into tediousness, I think it well to close my Narrative here. It has, in truth, already gone much beyond what I originally designed; and though I might have lengthened it yet further from my notes and recollections, and vivified it by more copious anecdotes, there is enough to satisfy the object for which I undertook it —that of leaving to my Children, and those who come in succession to them, such Memorial of my life as might serve for a family record hereafter, and furnish some motive and guidance to the latter—and perhaps to others also—in their progress through the world. Though devoid

of any important event, the incidents both of travel and
society have been sufficiently numerous and varied to
render such an epitome welcome even to myself for the
time that may yet remain to me. It rescues the *vita
anteacta* from that half-oblivion which time so generally
brings with it, overshadowing alike happy memories and
those of unhappiness. From the latter, as the preceding
Narrative will show, my own life has been singularly
exempt. The only causes of distress have been family
losses ; and öf these, for other reasons, I have spared
myself the record.

I have refrained also from mingling with my Narrative
any part of the political history of the time, except
where coming into connection with the persons or events
mentioned in it. I began life in what may be termed
the first year of the French Revolution. The eighty-
three years since elapsed have been prolific of changes
throughout the world at large—changes which deeply
concern the future destinies of mankind, and are ever
working towards unknown ulterior ends. Whatever these
may be, scarcely a year now passes without leaving a
certain mark behind it which time cannot efface. It is a
common thing to attach some epithet, rightly or wrongly,
to different ages in history. That we live in, may pre-
eminently be called an *age of transition.* What follows
after us must inevitably be different, and in many ways
widely contrasted with what has gone before.

But even had the design of this Volume been less
private and personal than it is, I should have refrained
from entering on these topics. The historians of the

period in which we live will be far more embarrassed by the multiplicity than by the paucity of the materials before them, and no contribution is needed to swell the amount. The talent of judicious selection will supersede that of recondite research ; while the philosophical historian will be called upon to review and record, not solely the results of wars, treaties, and party struggles, but also those more important and complex changes which political and physical science respectively have brought about in the social and national economy of the world. All speculations as to the future perfectibility of Man lie in this direction ; but with outlines dimly pictured even to the most prophetic eye.

A Roman poet has well said, ' It is living twice to be able to enjoy the past portion of life.' This expression, which I have willingly taken as the motto for my title-page, comes home to me as a present truth. I have been living again, and with enjoyment, while drawing upon these recollections of the past. Memories have been awakened which but for this motive to recall them would probably have slept on silently to the end of life. The occupation of reviving and reviewing these memories is one I do not willingly relinquish. They have even blended themselves agreeably and instructively with other enquiries to which I have devoted myself—those especially which regard the association of mental acts in their relation to time and sequence. The simple act of recalling an event which occurred sixty years before, is in itself the most wonderful of all phenomena. To discover the actual mechanism of this process, even in its simplest form, would be to gain the key to the inner-most mysteries of mental philosophy. But the problem is one which no research has hitherto solved, and pro-bably never will. It is a case where the confession of ignorance and inability becomes the truest philosophy.

Yet there are conditions, subordinate to this deeper problem, which come fairly within the scope of enquiry. The Memory, as represented in the ordinary occurrences of life, and still more as affected by accidents, disease, and old age, is in itself a great psychological volume—connecting, and in some sort embracing, all other mental phenomena. Facts, well attested, are here endless in number, and as strange as numerous; but I know no work which has duly systematised them. The treatise of Aristotle on Memory is almost as good as any of later times. Had I been younger, I should willingly have undertaken some such work; bringing in aid various notes derived from my own observation, and seeking for conclusions better defined than those we now possess; though still far short of any real comprehension of the mystery. I trust this object may hereafter be fulfilled by some one more capable than myself.

The Narrative which I here close, it is not likely I shall ever resume. Entering now on my eighty-fourth year, the changes and interests of the remainder of life must be chiefly, though not exclusively, such as regard my Children and Grandchildren, and therefore subject to those considerations which have led me to abstain from all family details. Were I ever to open again these pages of past life, it would probably be to amuse my leisure with some further scattered reminiscences of those various travels of which I have here given a slight and broken outline only. Such recollections may become a fair indulgence to a time when age or infirmity has brought to an end the faculty of travel itself, or needfully restricted it to some narrower circle around my own home.

LONDON : PRINTED BY
SPOTTISWOODE AND CO , NEW-STREET SQUARE
AND PARLIAMENT STREET